THE HEALTH
of the FAMILY *in a*
CHANGING ARABIA

THE HEALTH
of the FAMILY *in a*
CHANGING ARABIA

A CASE STUDY OF PRIMARY HEALTH CARE

ZOHAIR SEBAI

Professor of Family and Community Medicine

Second Edition

2014

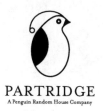

PARTRIDGE
A Penguin Random House Company

Library of Congress Control Number:		2014954928
ISBN:	Softcover	978-1-4828-2818-4
	eBook	978-1-4828-2819-1

To order additional copies of this book, contact
Toll Free 800 101 2657 (Singapore)
Toll Free 1 800 81 7340 (Malaysia)
orders.singapore@partridgepublishing.com

www.partridgepublishing.com/singapore

CONTENTS

LIST OF TABLES

LIST OF FIGURES

In the name of God, Most Gracious, Most Merciful

PREFACE

This study of health indicies and services in Turaba, Saudi Arabia was carried out in two stages. The author conducted the field research for his Doctorate degree in Public Health in Turaba in 1967 and this forms the basis of the second chapter of this book. For twelve years following 1969 he worked in the health field, as a planner, administrator and educator. During this period the author perceived that the primary health care system in Saudi Arabia (as well as in many other developing countries he visited) does not fulfill its potential role in promoting the health of the people.

During 1976 and 1981 the author returned to Turaba for two short visits to observe development in the health service system. He noted little change and his observations form the core material for the last two chapters.

In the author's opinion, the problem of primary care in Saudi Arabia, as could be the case in many other parts of the world, is related to the type of medical education and training received by physicians and other health personnel. In order to improve the primary Health Care System the starting point would be to modify the primary focus of medical education, emphasizing a community based, problem solving approach.

INTRODUCTION

S audi Arabia is a rapidly developing country with promising economic and human resources. From 1960 until 1980 (1380 –– 1400 A.H.) the health resources increased dramatically, well in excess of the population growth rate, particularly since 1974 (1394 A.H.).

Medical education in Saudi Arabia gives another perspective to the changes expected in the future. The graduates from the existing medical schools together with the medical students expected to qualify abroad, will increase the number of Saudi physicians from 460 in 1980 to an estimated 4,450 in 1995. By the year 2014 there became more than 15 medical schools and the number of the Saudi physicians exceeds 15,000.

The expansion of health services is taking place at all levels: primary, secondary and tertiary care. Primary health care has recently gained a great support with more centers to be established during the next ten years.

This study highlights the changes which have occurred in Turaba during the period 1967 - 1981. It presents us a lesson worth learning when planning for the future. The socio-economic development in this rural community has touched family life in many ways, seemingly carrying with it an improvement in health through better housing, nutrition and education.

Although the health center in Turaba was enlarged and its personnel increased during this period its function did not change, that of providing curative and palliative health services to the people. This is not a unique situation. Studies in several rural communities in the country in Asir[78], Hejaz[52] and Qasim[6][79] as well as in other neighboring Arab countries[76,77] showed the same pattern of health services. The problem looks more crucial if we consider that these types of Health Centers provide primary health care for more than 70% of the population.

The example of Turaba indicates that the expansion of health services by increasing the number of health units and personnel does not necessarily bring an improvement in health. The reasons are many: the knowledge and attitudes of the health personnel, determined largely by their hospital-based, curative-oriented medical education, the high percentage of non-Saudis (90% of the physicians and 80% of the paramedics) and the lack of orientation of the health workers to the ecology and health problems of the country.

The expansion of health services should be accompanied by a better understanding of the life style and set of values of the people, better knowledge of the health ecology, and better utilization of health resources, especially human.

This book offers a general framework of the development of primary health care in a rural community in Saudi Arabia, as well as in other Arab countries, based on the study of Turaba.

ACKNOWLEDGEMENTS

I would like to thank H.E. Sheikh Hasan Al El-Sheikh, and H.E. Sheikh Abdul Rahman Aba Al Khayl, whose assistance and support made this study possible.

I am indebted to the people of Turaba in general, and Sheikh Abdulla Al-Assaf, Sheikh Abdulla Bin Muhie and Sheikh Menahi Al Gharmool and the heads of the tribe in particular for their generosity which made our days in Turaba unforgettable.

I extend special thanks and appreciation to all my staff, interviewers, laboratory assistants and school teachers for their sincere help in the field.

I am also grateful to Dr. Timothy D. Baker, Professor of International health, for his continued advice during the early study.

Finally, I am indebted to my wife Ilham, whose loving encouragement, understanding and actual participation, were essential for bringing this study to its final form.

CHAPTER I

THE LAND AND THE PEOPLE

SAUDI ARABIA

Geography and People

On 18th September 1932, a royal decree was issued by King Abdul-Aziz Bin Saud, proclaiming the dual Kingdoms of Hejaz and Nejd to be unified under the new name, the Kingdom of Saudi Arabia. From the date of its establishment, Saudi Arabia has enjoyed full international recognition as an independent state.

The country occupies most of the Arabian Peninsula. It is bordered on the North by Jordan, Iraq and Kuwait, on the West by the Gulf of Aqaba and the Red Sea, on the South by Yemen Arab Republic and people's Democratic Republic of Yemen and on the East by Oman, Qatar, United Arab Emirates and the Arabian Gulf. The total land area is 2,149,000 km^2, which makes Saudi Arabia somewhat larger than England, France, Italy, Germany and Belgium combined.

The ancient Arabian shield protrudes eastward from Hejaz into Nejd as a bulge curving around from the Gulf of Aqaba to a point less than 200 km West of Riyadh and then receding toward the South near the Red Sea.

The largest desert area lies East of the shield. The great Nafud in the North and Rub'al Khali (the empty quarter) in the South are connected by the Dahana sand belt.

Arabia has one of the warmest climates in the world. The mean temperature is about 97°F in June and July; maximum temperatures of 118°F are recorded in the summer months. Winters are reasonably cool. The average annual rainfall throughout Arabia is generally very low, being 5 inches or less. The Asir Mountains Range in the South West is the only area in the Kingdom receiving adequate rainfall. The rest of the country is dry. Vegetation is sparse and widely scattered. The flora is also limited. The most important crops are dates, wheat, barley, corn and alfalfa. Fruits and vegetables are being grown in increasing amounts.

In 1980, the population of Saudi Arabia was estimated at 8.8 million. The estimated ratio of Bedouins varies, the most widely accepted figure is about 20%; apparently it is difficult to decide whether or not to include semi-settled people in this category. Arabs, like Europeans are largely of the Caucasian race. Bedouins are generally of the brown Mediterranean type. The population is predominantly Sunni Muslim mostly adhering to the Hanbali School of Islamic law. There is a minority of Shia, who live mainly in the Eastern Province.

Until 1926, when Ibn Saudi finally extended his domain over the whole of inner Arabia, the country had remained in almost total isolation from the rest of the world because of its poverty and arid land. Although the exploration for oil in the Eastern Province of Saudi Arabia began in early 1934, it was not drilled commercially until 1938. Suddenly, Saudi Arabia was catapulted into the Twentieth Century. The traditional, isolated, poor and mostly Bedouin country began to modernize. For the past 25 years, a progressive and persistent evolution has touched every aspect of life in Saudi Arabia. Culturally, socially and economically there have been changes, and more change is expected.

The settlement of Bedouins is one of the most prominent features of the development of the country. This settlement is accelerated by drought, social and geographic contact with the cities and the need for skilled labor for the newly emerging oil and mineral industries. There is very little available data about health conditions and associated socioeconomic factors of both nomadic and settled Bedouins.

Economy

The Kingdom produced 15.5% of the total world production of oil in 1980. The oil industry alone supplied 72.5% of the GDP. Saudi Arabia is economically stable and enjoys a strong foreign exchange position with a surplus balance of international payments. The GNP grew from SR. 6,543 million ($. 1,454 million) in 1965 to SR. 382 billion ($. 109 billion) in 1979. In 1979 the per capita income was estimated at SR. 43,000 ($. 12,300)[74] one of the highest in the world.

Development in the public sector has been focused on health, education, communications, agriculture, water resources and mineral deposits.

In the private sector the effort has been to encourage private investment and to attract outside expertise for industrialization.

Agriculture

Agriculture in Saudi Arabia faces many problems. Saudi Arabia is an inarable land which lacks perennial rivers. Only 0.23% of the total land is cultivated. Agriculture constitutes 1% of the GDP[84]. The total cultivated area of 592,000 hectares is worked by 600,000 workers, a low ratio of 0.987 hectares per worker.

Education

Education in Saudi Arabia has received major emphasis. In the 1960s the Ministry of Education promised the establishment of a primary school (which might be a classroom in a village or a settlement area) every third day. Every child is guaranteed free education to the limits of his abilities. There was, however, no obligation to remain at school to any predetermined age.

Between 1965 and 1980 the government educational budget increased from SR 408.3 million to SR 17.4 billion. The number of male students increased from 252,000 to 937,000 and the number of female students increased from 49,000 to 505,000.

Riyadh University, the first in the country, was established in 1957 with one college, the 'College of Arts'. By 1981 there were 7 universities with over 40 colleges. Between 1965 and 1980 the number of university students increased from 3,000 male and 66 female students to 36,000 and 13,100 respectively.

Because educational development in the Kingdom has occurred so recently, the majority of the adult population is understandably under-educated and under-trained.

Health Services

The health services system, from the time of its organization in 1950 through the late '60s, has developed slowly. However, during the last decade, the country has experienced a rapid expansion of all aspects of socio-economic life including the health services. The main factor behind this expansion was the substantial increase in the oil revenue of the country and the subsequent improvement in education, transport, communication, urbanization, Bedouin settlement and the inevitable increase in demand for health care.

The health problems in the Kingdom vary from communicable diseases such a malaria and schistosomiasis to those of a modern society with stress-related diseases, pollution and an ever increasing number of road accidents. With the country's vast economic resources many of its present health problems should soon come under control. The shortage of well-trained Saudi health personnel remains the principal difficulty.

The country is divided into 10 health regions each headed by a Regional Health Director. Most of the planning and decision making has been centralized in Riyadh, the capital. However regionalization has started with more authority being delegated to the Regional Directors.

Table 1 shows the distribution of the physical facilities in 1979. There are 14,200 beds i.e. 18 beds per 10,000 inhabitants (560 persons per bed), 380 Health centers and 506 dispensaries.

The expansion of the health services has depended primarily on expatriates, from Arab countries, Europe, USA, the Indian sub-continent and the Far East. The recruitment of large number of expatriates has helped in extending the services to every town and village in the country. However, the diversity of educational and cultural backgrounds has presented problems, as has the uneven urban-rural distribution and the main emphasis on curative medical care.

Almost 65% of all health personnel work in the Ministry of Health, 20% in other government agencies including the Military Services, Social Security, the Red Crescent, the National Guard, School Health, the Department of Girls Education and the municipalities, and 15% in the private sector.

At present there are 5,300 physicians working in Saudi Arabia. 60% being general practitioners, the remainder are specialists holding 2––4 year diplomas. There is an uneven distribution of physicians. Most of them work in the 96 hospitals and 447 private clinics located in cities.

Most of the physicians have been trained in clinically oriented, hospital-based institutions which emphasize physician-patient relationships. Many of the physicians and other health personnel lack adequate knowledge of the ecology of health and disease and of the socio-economic and cultural background of Saudi society.

Out of the total number of physicians, there are 460 Saudi nationals (9%). The output of the four Medical Schools in Saudi Arabia is expected to reach 3,130 physicians by the turn of the decade with another 1,300 physicians expected to graduate from abroad.

Table 2 shows the ratio of Saudis to the total health manpower. Until recently most of the expatriates came from Egypt, India and Pakistan. More recruitment is now being carried out in Britain, USA and the Far East. Because of the difficulties faced in running some of the new modernized hospitals, complete teams were recruited from the USA, Denmark and Taiwan.

The total number of physicians trained in public health does not exceed 100. Most of them are administrators. Only 5 Saudi physicians have received formal training in public health.

In 1977 there were 9,900 health assistants of whom 46% were female nurses, 18% male nurses and 36% technical assistants. 22% were Saudi (only 7% of the female nurses were Saudi). Most of the expatriate health assistants were recruited from Egypt, Pakistan and India. Increasing numbers are being recruited from the Philippines and from South Korea.

In order to increase the number of Saudi health personnel, four Medical Schools, a Faculty of Dentistry, a Faculty of Health Sciences, a Faculty of Veterinary Medicine and a Department of Hospital Administration were established between 1969 and 1980. A Faculty of Public Health is now being planned in the University of Riyadh.

There are 3 Health Institutes to train male health assistants and 7 Nursing Schools to train female nurses.

An effort is being made to revise the curricula in the three established Medical Schools, and to establish a new program in the fourth Medical School in Abha.. The object is to produce physicians appropriately trained to function as members of the health team and capable of meeting the health needs of the country. Steps have already been taken towards integrated teaching and community-based training.

Table - 1
Distribution of hospitals, beds and ambulatory care units according to sector (1979).

	Hospitals	Hospital Beds	Clinics	Health Centers	Dispensaries
Ministry of Health	70	10,412	––	299	506
Other Govt. Organizations	11	2,605	––	81	––
Private Sector	15	1,183	447		––
Total:	96	14,200	447	380	506

A H.C. is run by physicians while a dispensary is run by a health assistant.

Table - 2
Percentage of Saudi Personnel (1980)

	Total	Saudi No.	%
Physicians	5.300	460	9
Dentists	280	30	11
Health Assistants	12,800	2,700	21

TURABA

Geography

Turaba is an area of approximately 18,500 sq km in West Saudi Arabia (Figure 1). It extends about 90 km from the North at Shir to the South at Khyala. In the East it extends to Harat Turaba and in the West to Jabal Hadn, an important historical landmark, separating Najd from Hejaz.

In the middle of the area lie two wadis (valleys), "Wadi Turaba" and "Wadi Kara". They run from the South to the north parallel to each other, until they meet 15 km from the Northern border of Turaba. The old volcanic area between the two wadis is 6 km at its widest part. The cultivated area is surrounded and intermingled by grazing areas and barren land, and fed by underground water through several hundred shallow dug wells and water holes.

History

Turaba, like many other parts in the country, has an old culture, as indicated by a ruin of an ancient city 2 km South of Souq, the main town. Our team found pre-Islamic pottery in the ruins. We also discovered a Neolithic flint point in the stone desert in the north.

In recent history; Turaba held a strategic position at the side of Jabal Hadan, a natural landmark between Najd and Hejaz. Because of this, it was the scene of many battles. The last battle was in 1918 (1337 A.H.) between King Abdul Aziz troops sweeping from Najd towards Hejaz and the troops of Hashemite in Turaba. The victory of Saudi troops in Turaba was a decisive one and in a few years King Abdul Aziz swept from Turaba to Taif and Mecca and took over Hejaz.

Administration

Before the different parts of the Kingdom were united by the late King Abdul Aziz, every tribe was practically governed by itself. Often a sub-tribe emerged as a single entity and formed an independent tribe. As a result, wars and battles between and within the tribes extended through the whole history of the area. When the strong man, Abdul Aziz, came, he put an end to the tribal conflicts.

Turaba is governed now by the "Emir of Turaba", who is responsible to the "Emir of Mecca", the governor of the Western region of the country The latter, in turn, is responsible to the Minister of the Interior.

Problems ranging from a case of divorce to a big conflict within the tribe are dealt with first by the heads of the tribe and the old members of the community. If they cannot solve the problem, it is referred to the judge "Kadi" in Souq, who is the judicial authority in Turaba. His decision is final in most cases and the Emir of Turaba executes the verdict. If the party is not satisfied, he might complain to the Emir of Mecca, the Minister of the Interior, or the King himself. The heads of the tribes and sub-tribes have a traditionally honored position which helps to solve most of the problems.

People and Community

The area is inhabited mostly by the Begum Tribe, one of the major tribes in Saudi Arabia. The tribe is divided into two main branches — "Wazi" and Mahamid" — and each branch divided into 14 sub-division "Fakhdh" (Figure 2). Some "Fakhdh" of the tribes are traced to different areas in the country, even to al Rub al Khali "Empty Quarter".

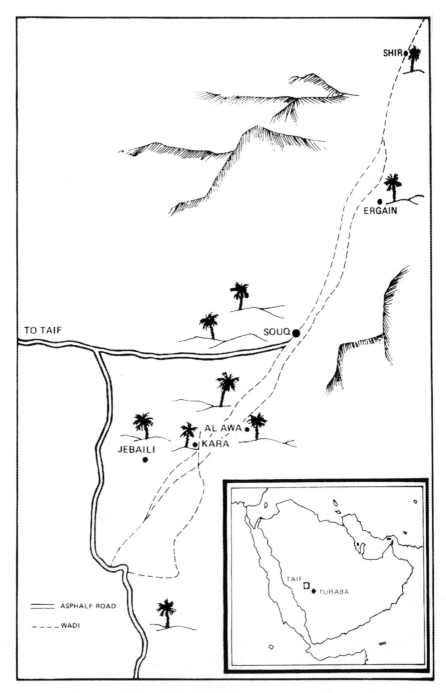

Figure 1. Map of Wadi Turaba – the area of the study.

There is no accurate census of the population of Turaba; however it was estimated at 30,000 in 1967 and 45,000 in 1981. The population dynamic is a combination of a natural growth (about 2.8 per year), settlement of Bedouin tribes from outside Turaba migration to cities and the importation of expatriates, mostly unskilled laborers, for farming.

The population is of three types.

1. Settled –– with a history of settlement over 25 years. They live primarily in the two main towns of Souq and Alawa. Their main occupations are government employment, trade and some farming. In general they enjoy a better economy than the rest of the tribe and have ready access to health services.

2. Semi-settled –– with a history of settlement of less than 20 years. They live mostly in settlement areas "Hejrat" scattered along the two wadis of Turaba. They practice agriculture and some animal husbandry.

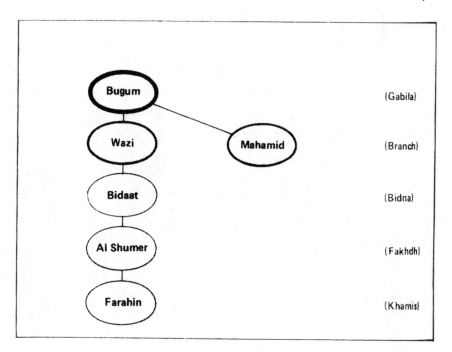

Figure 2. The Branches of Bugum Tribe.

3. Nomadic Bedouins — they are still nomadic with no fixed residence. They seasonally wander from place to place, within a defined territory. They all live in tents and their main source of income is animal husbandry.

The proportion of population of each type, the style of life, type of housing, education and other features, have changed in the past fifteen years.

Settlement of Bedouins has developed rapidly, mostly because of the drought and the improved economy of settled life. The estimated proportion of nomads decreased from 30% in 1967 to less than 20% in 1981. According to a United Nations Report, "the last nomadic Bedouin will pack his tent and migrate to the city by 1995".

Villages

Souq is the oldest village, located in the center of Turaba and considered as its administrative capital. It contains the Emir house, other government offices, the Development Center and the main market of Turaba. The estimated population (1980) is 9,000. Seventy per cent come from the Bugum Tribe, predominantly the branch of Mahamid. The remaining thirty percent are foreign expatriates Negroes and tribe less migrants from the cities. Souq is connected by a 140 km asphalted road to Taif City, (approx. 250,000 population), the summer capital of the government.

Alawa is the second most important village after Souq and lies 5 km south of Souq. The approximate 5,000 inhabitants are mainly from the "Wazi" branch of the tribe. About 8% of the people are Ashraf, descendants of the prophet Mohammed. Alawa village alone has about 20% of the cultivated area of Turaba.

Settlement Areas (Hejar)

Settlement areas were established during the last 50 years. The name "hejar" was given first by the late King Abdul Aziz, who started the process of Bedouin settlement in 1911. One of the first "Hejar" established at that time was "Hejrat Bani Ghannam", in Turaba in the 1940s. By 1965 there were eleven "hejar" and by 1981 the number of "hejar" grew to 26 with almost double the number of population. The "hejar" vary in size, from "Absia" (60 households), to "Ergain" (above 200 households).

The inhabitants of the "hejar" are more homogeneous than those in villages in the sense that they are predominantly from one Fakhdh.

There might be some expatriate laborers who work temporarily in house construction and farming, but no negro or Ashraf, and seldom members of another tribe.

The selection of the area of the settlement is usually made by the old wise men of the sub-tribe. Sheikh Minahi says, "I touched the land, inspected the branches of the Wadi, the sloping mountains around and then said to my people, here will you grow palm trees, onions and wheat". A few pioneers from the group settle down, followed gradually over the years by others. The whole process is usually managed by the head of the sub-tribe. He divides the land among the newcomers, according to their position in the tribe and the size of their families. Usually a line of demarcation separates the settlement areas of the different parties.

The government encourages the process of settlement by helping in reclamation of the land and by providing the farmers with machinery, seeds, fertilizers, financial loans and other agricultural assistance. Whenever disagreements arise between two sub-tribes about the natural boundaries between their territories, the government takes **over** the whole territory and sells it at symbolic prices to the members of the involved groups.

In Hejar people grow mainly palm trees, and some vegetables and citron trees. Some of them raise goats and sheep as an additional source of income. In these settlement areas, the original traditional black tents made of goats hair changed gradually over the years into huts and mud houses and recently into block and concrete buildings. The proportion of each differs according to the time elapsed and to the degree of settlement. The main markets for Turaba produce are Mecca and Taif. Besides that, Turaba is an important source of citron for Hejaz. However, most of the villages and settlement areas are greatly affected by drought.

Nomadic Bedouins

Nomadic Bedouins in Turaba live in black tents and raise goats, sheep and to a lesser extent, camels. Their main grazing areas are Khyala and Elaba, 50 km South of Souq; Jabal Hadn, 40 km Northwest of Souq; and Riyadh Bani Ghannam, 140 km North of Souq.

In the winter (the rain season), nomads live in small groups (3––10 tents) widely separated, where their animals can graze freely. In the summer, when there is no rain or grass, they gather round water holes in groups of 30––50 tents. The very old traditional system (Al Hema) where a tribe or even a sub-tribe sticks to its own grazing land has been abrogated by the government. However, it is still traditionally observed. The movement of the Bedouins became very limited in the last decade due to the drought and other factors (see Chapter III).

CHAPTER II

TURABA
THE PAST 1967

METHODOLOGY

In the summer of 1966, I left John Hopkins University, Baltimore for Saudi Arabia to conduct a pilot study for the field work of my doctorate degree in Public Health.

During the four month period of the pilot study, I conducted small-scale surveys in seven different communities (Figure 3). In the meantime, I met authorities from different ministries and agencies.

Turaba, among other areas, stood out as the most suitable place for the study:

1. It combined three communities of different stages of settlement —— settled, semi-settled and nomads.

2. Sheikhs of the tribe and the Emir of Turaba were very cooperative and willing to have the study undertaken in Turaba.

3. The Development Center, a prominent feature in Turaba, was one of 17 centers established during the 1960s in the country 'to uplift social, economic and education aspects with the cooperation and participation of the natives'. The health division, one of the four divisions in the Development Center, was staffed by a Pakistani doctor and five paramedical personnel. The Development Center promised to provide personnel, accommodation and laboratory facilities (electricity, refrigerator, running water and laboratory space).

In the early summer of 1967, I left Baltimore for the second time for Saudi Arabia, to conduct the main study.

The hypothesis was that in Wadi Turaba there were no significant differences in the health status of children of 0—4 years old in settled, semi-settled and nomadic communities.

This hypothesis has been based on a series of observations made during the pilot study. The conclusions of these observations were:

1. There is not much difference in health knowledge, attitude or practice between settled, semi-settled and nomadic Bedouins.

2. The Health Center activities which are accessible to the settled population do not seem to have had much influence on the health of the people.

The objectives of the field work were then defined as:

1. To determine the health status of children 0—4 years of age in selected settled, semi-settled and nomadic communities.

2. To identify the socio-economic and environmental factors and available health services which might influence the children's health condition in each community.

The survey was planned to include about 300 households selected at random in communities with different stages of settlement. The elements of the study were to include closed and open-ended questionnaires to the households, clinical, anthropometric and laboratory examinations for pre school children and the study of certain socio-economic aspects and the health services systems available to the communities.

Sample Size

Because of the time available for the study, the number of the personnel and the type of the community, we planned to study 300 households. Actually, we ended up studying 314 households in six different localities and reinterviewed 20% of those who were interviewed (Table 3). Th ramifications of the sample size are shown in the Appendix.

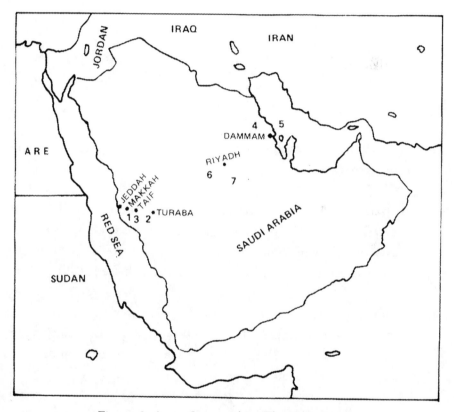

Figure 3. Areas Surveyed In The Pilot Study

LEGEND

1. WADI FATIMA
2. WADI TURABA
3. SHAFA MOUNTAIN
4. VILLAGE OF SAFWA

5. ISLAND OF TARUT
6. KABSHAN AREA
7. VILLAGE OF HYATHEM

Table - 3
Areas of the study, their distances from Souq and number of households studied.

Area	Distance from Souq in k. m.	Mud	Households Hut	Studied Tent	Total
Souq	––	87	––	––	87
Kara	18	48	22	17	87
Ergain	27	23	4	32	59
Alawa	4	––	––	13	13
Jebaili	8	7	13	28	48
Elaba	40	––	3	17	20
		165	42	107	314

Our Sample was divided into three groups (communities) A, B and C according to the degree of settlement.

Community A –– 87 Households: A settled community, all living in Souq. The majority of people have a settlement history of more than 10 years. All are living in mud houses. They have better economic status and more accessibility to health services through the Health Center.

Community B –– 120 Households: A semi-settled community. They live in mud houses and huts outside Souq. The majority have settlement history of less than 7 years. They depend on farming as the main source of income.

Community C –– 107 Households: A nomadic community. They are still nomads, live in tents, with no fixed residence, but seasonally wander from place to place within a defined territory. Their main source of income is husbandry.

(The notation Communities A, B and C is used for all subsequent tables).

Personnel

Our team, composed of 21 persons, was based in the Development Center. The survey 'activities' covered 314 families living in the main village, Souq, and 5 other settlement and Bedouin areas. We stayed in Turaba for three months from July through September 1967. The number and type of personnel who participated in the study were as follows:

Number	Type of Personnel	
1	main investigator	
4	female interviewers	1 nurse, 2 social workers and the investigator's wife.
5	male interviewers	3 social workers and 2 local teachers.
2	laboratory assistants	from Ministry of Health
1	clerk	from the community.
2	Khawi	Emir representatives.
4	female companions	hired locally.
2	drivers	

Male and female interviewers were trained separately. In the first few days, training was held in the office. Thoughtful explanation and discussion of every item in the questionnaire was carried out. Under observation and guidance, interviewers interviewed each other. Male and female patients from the out-patient department in the Health Center were asked to participate as interviewees. Then a village, Quaia, 8 km from Souq, not intended to be included in the study, was selected for field training. The period of training took 12 days.

Elements of the study

I. The Questionnaire

A. Close-ended questionnaire

i) **Face Sheet**
Carried out by the male interviewers with the heads of the households. Areas covered were: demographic data, household members, number, age, sex, marital status, education and whether any child had been born in the household in the last five years. Subsequently every household with a child born in the last five years was included in the study.

ii) **Mother Questionnaire**
Carried out by the female interviewers with the mothers. Areas covered were: history of morbidity, history of pregnancy and its outcome, knowledge, attitudes and practice of family planning and nutrition of the family and the child.

iii) **Child Questionnaire**
Carried out by the female interviewers (at the same sitting as the mother questionnaire) with the mothers of children 0—4 years old. Areas covered were: history of morbidity and treatment, accidents, immunization and weaning.

iv) **Head of Household Questionnaire**
Carried out by the male interviewers with the heads of the households. Areas covered were: history of morbidity, health knowledge, attitude and practice, economic status, history of settlement, health demands and environmental sanitation.

The questionnaires were designed in English, discussed and then translated into Arabic. They were tested twice (in Turaba and Wadi Fatima) before they were finally printed, semi-coded in classic Arabic. The local dialect is closer to classic Arabic than the dialect spoken in some other parts of the country or other Arab countries.

We constructed a Calendar of Events to determine the age of children below five years. The main elements of the calendar were: Exactly at two years of age, each child is weaned (unless the mother is pregnant, then the child will be weaned earlier). Ramadan and Al Haj are the two holy months in which people fast or pilgrim to Mecca. Al Geedha is the season of harvesting the date, in which almost all the people participate directly or indirectly. The recent big events in Turaba were the flood, the big quarrel between members of Al Rahamen sub-tribe, the assignment of the director of the Development Center and the new judge.

B. Open-ended Questionnaire

I carried most of this part out with well-informed people (key informants) in Turaba, mainly at the end of the study. The meetings, friendly and informal, were mostly held in the homes of the people. Coffee, tea, dates and milk and frequently the traditional food of a Bedouin to his guest –– meat and rice –– were served during the interviews. Notes were taken without objections.

The areas covered were a wide range of social, cultural, economic, dietary and environmental aspects of life. The persons and places were chosen independently from those included in the close-ended study.

II. Clinical, Anthropometric and Laboratory Examinations

In the first four weeks of the study mothers and children were brought by the landrover vehicle to the Health Center for clinical and laboratory examinations. We found it more practical and convenient to the people to move with the essential laboratory equipment to the area of study. People became more interested in the study since we were able to provide them with treatment for their mild ailments and participation in the clinical and laboratory tests increased. One of the houses in the center of the community, usually the sheikh's house, was selected for the purpose.

Children and adults were treated for simple ailments. Whenever an elaborate history and physical examination was required, the case referred to the Health Center. Often one of the two cars was provided for transportation of the sick.

A. Clinical Examination

Every participating child was examined clinically. Certain clinical signs were selected to assess nutritional and disease conditions.

B. Anthropometric Measurements

Children, after the clinical examination, were referred to the male nurse to measure their weight, height, head circumference and chest circumference. The Standard UNICEF balance scale was used for weighing young children, and a regular platform balance scale was used for weighing the older ones. Head and chest measurements were done by a flexible non-stretch tape on the levels of the maximum occipital prominences and the nipple line. Children were examined and measured nude except for a light covering for older girls.

C. Laboratory Work

Finally, the child was referred to the laboratory assistant to collect material; blood for haemoglobin, malaria and serological tests; stools; and rectal swabs. Some of the laboratory processes such as separation and preservation of the sera, preparation of the malaria smears, and haemoglobin readings were done in the field.

Serum samples and rectal swab specimens were shipped by plane in dry ice to the Communicable Disease Center in Atlanta, Georgia, for bacteriological and virological studies. Stool and malaria specimens were examined in the Department of Pathobiology, The John Hopkins School of Public Health and Hygiene, Baltimore.

Problems encountered during the study:

Intravenous Blood

At the beginning of the study, intravenous blood was used for the various blood tests. By the end of the second week, we realized that the people had a strong feeling against withdrawing blood from the children. The loss of blood means loss of power and strength. The reaction was so severe that it affected the degree and quality of participation in both the questionnaire and the clinical and laboratory tests.

Rumors started to spread that we were using the blood for our own purposes. Some of the rumors said that we were using "the power in the blood" by adding it to our tea. Since we were substituting tea for water, this rumor appeared to have a concrete basis. Others said that were selling the blood to the Blood Bank in Mecca. A third group said that we were analyzing their children's blood in order to select them for the army when they came of age.

Lack of Understanding

The idea of the study was never clear enough in the minds of the people. From the early beginning, it was realized that any scientific explanation of the purpose of the study would not be accepted or even understood. People in Turaba, as everywhere, are interested in solutions for their problems rather than being used as a study group. They were looking for something positive to be done for them.

Their health demands are simple. They want a Health Center or dispensary, injections and a doctor or a nurse to take care of their sick. At the beginning they could not see a relationship between what they wanted and our questions about family planning and health knowledge, attitudes and practices.

The Bedouin believes that he is more intelligent than most of the city people and the questionnaire were considered a challenge to his intelligence. He must know in exact, simple, straightforward words why we are here and what we are doing, otherwise he will not cooperate. His sheikh may persuade him to participate in a certain activity, but he can never force him to do it. Most of the people in Turaba are either Bedouin or of Bedouin descent.

Our approach to the community was formulated in a simple way. "The government is interested in the improvement of your health conditions. We are here to study your problems and how we can solve them. Afterwards, we will report to the government, and there is nothing more we can do. The government will decide what to do".

They always believe in the central government, which put an end to their constant inter-tribal wars and established justice, and they were satisfied with the frank statement about our purpose. However, they were motivated in some areas of the study by their own experience that surveys are connected to social welfare assistance. Examples of these areas are their distorted responses to the questionnaire about their incomes, food consumption and the age of the head of the family.

Inter-tribal Conflicts

The Bugum Tribe is divided into 28 sub-tribes (Fakhdh) and each sub-tribe is composed of several groups (Khamis).

Conflict may occur every now and then between different sub-tribes or even between different "Khamis" within the same sub-tribe. Most conflicts occur due to claims for a piece of land or a nomadic range. Careful approaches were used whenever two neighboring conflicting parties were under study.

An example of this is in Esala where a recent conflict divided the Groof Khamis into two parties, separated by Wadi Turaba. When we started the study, we began the enumeration and the demographic survey from the West of the Wadi, proceeding to the East. This resulted in the enragement of the Sheikh of the group living in the East of the Wadi. To satisfy him, we selected his house for the clinical and laboratory work, but the other group was not satisfied. When the Eastern group invited the laboratory workers for a lamb, the other group invited the whole team for a two-lamb lunch the next day. More time was spent in the area than was originally planned, in order to satisfy both parties.

Despite these minor conflicts, the people of Turaba during the last half century have experienced the most peaceful period in their history. Under the strong Saudi rule the previously persistent wars between and within the tribes have come to an end.

SOCIO-ECONOMIC

ECONOMY

Sources of Income

The main sources of income in Turaba are occupation, relatives working in cities, rafda, and furga.

Occupation: Table 4 shows the occupations of the heads of the households as it was elicited by interviewing.

Table - 4
Percent distribution of heads of households by occupation

Com.	Resp.	None	Farmer	Herds man	Employee or Merchant	Soldier	Non Skilled Laborer	Other	Total
A	58	5	5	—	61	5	18	6	100
B	106	2	67	3	2	13	8	5	100
C	88	9	28	36	1	7	10	9	100

Sixty-one per cent of the people in Souq enjoy the stable and relatively high income of government employment and commerce. Only 5 per cent mentioned farming as the main occupation. Actually, most of the merchants, and to a lesser extent the employees, have their own land either in Souq or Alawa, cultivated by hired laborers. Those listed as soldiers work in the army, mainly in Riyadh or Taif, but were vacationing with their families in Turaba.

Farming is the main occupation of the semi-settled people (67 per cent). With the prevalent drought, most of the land is, unfortunately, not productive. According to Italian Council*, in 1958 the cultivated area in Turaba was 609 hectares. In 1965 it dropped to 420 hectares.

Livestock is the main source of income for the nomadic people. However, usually the children and the young adults take care of the sheep herding.

In the studied nomadic group some of the heads of the households were hired in the two-month summer period for harvesting the dates. A few of them started to cultivate, unsuccessfully, small plots around their water holes. A total of 28 per cent reported farming as their main occupation. I noted that it appears more prestigious for the nomads to mention (farming), and also it indicates a general trend for settlement.

Relatives working in the cities: Almost every family in the nomadic and semi-settled communities has a member who is working in the city and helping support the family financially. Most of the working members join the white army (National Guard). A few of them join the police force or hold a small position in the government. Very few have private jobs or work in merchandising. Practically none work as tailors, butchers, or bakers, which, according to the standards of the tribe, are not respectable jobs.

There are two main reasons for the great tendency to join the army –– one is the possibility of receiving a regular education up to the sixth grade or higher, and the other is the similarity to the natural life of the Bedouin as guardians of the camp and livestock**.

---

* An Italian company surveying the country for water and soil resources for the Ministry of Agriculture.
** Aramco Oil Company in Dhahran has found that most of the Bedouin employees prefer driving or jobs related to security

In Riyadh I tried to get statistical figures from the National Guard headquarters concerning the number and percentage of people from Turaba joining the National Guard, but no statistics were available.

Rafda: A needy man who does not have a relative to support him may go and ask for help from his tribal men working in the city. There is no feeling of begging or charity in this act, but rather a feeling of rights and obligations. A man might pay two or three visits every year to the cities. Every time he might be able to visit about five persons, and he might collect about SR. 40 from each.

Fugra. In cases of disaster, every man in the tribe is responsible for his fellow man. At the time we were in Turaba we experienced a very tragic accident in which a school boy was run over by a truck. For years the quiet valley of Turaba had not seen such an accident. The boy's father had the right to get "Al Dia", which is SR. 16,000 ($. 3,300) paid by the driver; otherwise the latter would be in jail, perhaps for life. The family of the driver borrowed the money from one of the merchants in Souq and gave it to the boy's father in a ceremony "to forgive". Then it was the responsibility of some delegated members of the tribe to collect the SR. 16,000 from all people in the tribe, which happened to include close relatives of the killed boy. In about six weeks the whole amount was collected and repaid to the merchant.

Economic Status

Various methods were adopted to study the economic status of the people under the study: (1) the questionnaire — heads of the households were asked about their income, expenditures and owned tangible wealth; (2) the interviewers as well as key informants estimated the economic status of the households.

Income and expenditure: Table 5 shows the monthly income per household in the three areas, as it was elicited by the questionnaires.

Table - 5
Percent distribution of households by monthly income in Saudi Riyals

Com.	Resp.	200	201–500	500+	Total	Measuring Scale
A	57	32	51	17	100	10.1
B	106	86	14	–	100	5,7
Could	86	93	6	1	100	5.4

Measuring scale: A constant value is attached to each category.

SR. < 200 = 0.5
SR.   201–500 = 1
SR. > 500 = 2

Throughout the study it was noticed that in most nomadic and semi-settled communities, the expenditure was stated as being higher than the income. At that time I felt it was a nuisance to collect such information. The only reason I kept collecting the data was that I was interested in this difference between income and expenditure. In the analytic stage, I found that only among the low income group (SR. < 200) was the expenditure stated higher than the income. My interpretation for this is, the people, particularly the poor in nomadic and semi-settled communities, always associated our study with the social welfare assistance given by the government. Consequently, they tend most of the time to underestimate their income and overestimate their expenditure to prove they are needy. It is interesting to note that in overestimating their expenditures, they very seldom exceed a certain limit (SR. 200), at which they feel they would be satisfied.

Tangible wealth: Another criterion, tangible wealth, was used beside monthly income and expenditure, to assess the difference in economic status of families in the three communities. Five items, gasoline lamp, radio, sewing machine, stove, and pressure lantern, were selected, and the interviewee was asked whether he owned them or not. (Table 6).

There is an apparent difference between the three communities in owning the five items. This difference is confirmed statistically (P = .005). We found that the tangible wealth in this case could be taken as a more sensitive and meaningful index of wealth than income and expenditure. However, we should consider that a wealthy nomad might spend his money on slaughtering more sheep for his guests rather than buying a radio or a stove.

Table - 6

Percent distribution of households possessing certain items of tangible wealth.

Com.	Resp.	None	Gasoline Lamp	Radio	Sewing Machine	Stove	Pressure Lantern	All Items*
A	56	0	22	68	66	70	70	43
B	102	2	81	20	17	6	11	3
C	59	10	51	12	8	5	8	2

Interviewer's estimate: Male interviewers and selected key informers were asked to record their impression of the economic status of the household in one of the three grades: affluent, average, or poor. There was no definite or standardized criterion for this evaluation, just the personal impression reflected by the appearance of the individual and the house, its contents, furniture and surroundings:

Measuring scale: There is an apparent agreement between the scales of income, expenditure and the interviewers' and key informants estimation in the three communities. Community A had almost double the scale of B and C. Semi-settled is always higher than nomadic, but the difference is slight.

Conclusion: With the previously presented data, we do not pretend that we have the most sensitive or accurate index of the economic status of the people under the study. I can say, however, that it reflects a picture of the situation.

---

*   Except gasoline lamp.

In Souq the employees gave their exact incomes and the merchants averaged theirs. The soldiers, as well, gave their exact income. The unskilled laborers, although they were not precise about the number of days they worked per month, still mentioned their daily wages. For the farmers, and more so for the pastoral workers, a regular fixed monthly or even yearly income does not exist. Their expenditures vary from time to time. The estimates they gave of their monthly income and expenditure was not far from reality. Apart from distortion from hopes of social welfare assistance, there was no problem in collecting the data. There was no fear of taxation, which is practically nil, if any. Al Zakat (alms-giving) is usually left to the people to give on their own.

We might conclude that from the data collected, we found an apparent difference between the economic status of Souq and the other two communities.

Among the various socio-economic parameters we have studied, I believe that this difference in the economic status of the two populations plays the greatest role in determining the health condition of the children. For some time researchers have been interested in the interrelationship between economic status and health conditions of a population.

On a national level and in case studies of Chile and Puerto Rico the author concluded, "Health services alone do not provide an effective measure of improving health. Economic welfare is the most important factor in improving levels of health".[53]

In the U.S. National Health Survey of 80,000 male workers in eight American cities, it was found that families with incomes below $. 1,000 per year had 66 per cent more sickness and disability than the families with incomes over $. 5,000[88].

On the international level, the United Nations in their report on the world social situation[87], classified seventy countries into six groups according to the national per capita income. In the report it was shown that per capita income is closely related to the level of education (percentage of school population), nutritional status (calorie intake per day), infant mortality rate, and life expectancy at birth in years.

Here we can best conclude with a quote from Baker[5], "Economic level per se has no direct causal relationship with morbidity, but acts through a series of more or less closely correlated variables, such as age, sex, health practices, nutrition, housing, availability of medical care, and so forth".

In our study, many of the previously mentioned variables correlated with the health condition of the three communities, will be discussed later.

SOCIAL LIFE

Settlement

"The project of Bedouin settlement is one of the most complicated processes which aims for the development and life improvement of a part of the human race". Filali[*22]

The seasonal movement of nomadic tribes —— determined by supplies of water and pasture —— has become very limited in Turaba in the last seven years due to the drought. Many of the nomads did not exceed a radius of ten miles in their seasonal movements in the last two years.

Settlement of nomads is increasingly accelerated. In Esala, for example, twenty families, out of a total eighty households, settled in the last year, and the trend is continuing. We asked 144 persons in Communities A and B, who have been nomads in the past, about the reason for their settlement (Table 7).

---

*   M. Filali, a previous Minister of Agriculture in Tunisia was assigned by the Saudi Arabian government to study nomadism in the country. Unpublished data.

Table - 7

**Reasons for settlement of people in communities
A and B with history of nomadism.**

Com.	Resp.	Cause of Settlement			
		Drought		Other	
		No.	%	No.	%
A	23	10	44	13	56
B	121	93	77	28	24

It appears that most people (56 per cent) in Souq have settled because of reasons other than drought. They settled gradually over several decades. On the other hand, semi-settled people in Community B settled, in general, because of the drought (77 per cent).

Settlement appears to be more promising and more comfortable. Among those who had a history of nomadism in Communities A and B, 119 were asked whether they would go back to nomadic life if the rain come back. Only five said yes; the remaining (114) said no. The reasons for that are:

Number	Reason
37	no animals
11	tired of nomadism
49	want settlement
13	other reasons
4	no reason
—————	
114	Total

On all counts nomadism is a tough life. Even though at the time of rains (Al Haia = Life) there is plenty of meat, milk and butter, few of those who have settled would go back to nomadism if the rains came back.

Concept of Nomadism and Settlement: Heads of the households were asked about the advantages and disadvantages of nomadism and settlement.

Advantage of settlement (Table 8): Comfort was valued very highly among people in the three communities. No doubt, nomadism, especially with the drought, is a very hard and subsistance level of life. Availability of money was valued next by semi-settled and nomads. Health and education were valued low among all, although the health centers and the school are among the first priorities for Bedouins.

Advantage of nomadism over settlement: Sentimental values such as hospitality, neighborliness', braveness and morality, are the main characteristics which the Bedouins of the desert still have, and they are proud of it. Dickson[12] said, "Every Bedouin, whether rich or poor, must entertain and feed a stranger who asks for a night's lodging". He mentioned a story about the late King Abdul Aziz. "It has been addressed to me in my capacity as guest on several occasions, notably by H.M. King King Abdul Aziz Al Saud when I visited him in 1920. "O, guest of ours, though you have come, though you have visited us, and though you have honored our dwellings, we verily are the real guests and you are the lord of this house". "Walpole[90] mentioned that the Bedouins consider themselves to be the purest of the Arabs. They are proud of their heritage and their way of life as it is celebrated in poetry and legends.

Table - 8
Percent distribution of perceived advantages of settlement over nomadism.

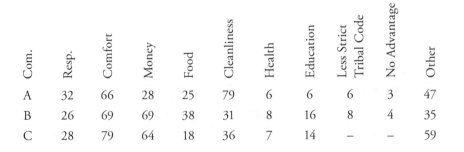

Com.	Resp.	Comfort	Money	Food	Cleanliness	Health	Education	Less Strict Tribal Code	No Advantage	Other
A	32	66	28	25	79	6	6	6	3	47
B	26	69	69	38	31	8	16	8	4	35
C	28	79	64	18	36	7	14	–	–	59

If a villager is poor, nobody will care for him. More respondents said there is no advantage in nomadism than those who said there is no advantage in settlement.

Settlement of nomads is a natural process which has been enhanced in the last decade by the drought and cultural contacts with the cities. According to Saber7 3, "The desert is not and never was a constant fact neither in time nor in place, and the change is going on". He foresees that one day nomadism will become a historical phenomenon.

Two main problems are facing the sudden process of settlement in Turaba now:

1. Bedouins are not experienced in agriculture, and there is a scarcity of water.

2. The sudden change might affect the social and cultural values as well as the family and kinship ties.

The government is accelerating settlement and more planning is proposed for the process.

Migration

The young people of Turaba usually migrate at the age of eighteen, the age of acceptance in the army. In many instances, the migration starts at an earlier age, around ten years, if the child has a brother or a cousin in the city with whom he can stay to attend school. The scarcity of the young generation in the Bedouin communities is a striking feature; one can seldom find a young man 15 to 25 years old.

In the army a young soldier from Turaba starts at a salary of about SR 250 (U.S. $. 55/month). While he builds up his own family –– mostly he marries from Turaba –– his salary goes up steadily. He sends back about 25 to 30 per cent of his salary to his family in Turaba.

Literacy

A sample of adult couples (heads of households and their wives) were asked about their ability to read and write. The percentage of respondents claiming literacy is shown in Table 9. The literacy among males and females in Souq is high compared to both sexes in the other two communities. This difference may be reflected in their concept of health and diseases and, consequently, on their children's health status.

Table - 9
Percent distribution of literacy amongst heads
of households and their wives.

Community	Heads	% Literate	Wives	% Literate
A	86	39	84	7
B	121	15	121	0.8
C	99	4	101	0.9

However, this is a sample of an old generation. Education is highly valued now in all communities. Schools are one of the first priorities among all. Migration of young men to cities is motivated largely by seeking education, mostly in the army. Girls' education is increasingly accepted in Souq. Among nomads, girls' education is still not fully accepted "unless others get their girls educated".

The Family

Structure and dynamics. Social relations in Saudi Arabia are directly or indirectly tied to family considerations. The family is the fundamental and essential repository of every indivudual's personal identity. Patai[61] describes the traditional Middle East family as characterized by the following six traits: extended, patrilineal, patrilocal, patriarchal, endogenous, and occasionally polygamous. Most of these traits, if not all of them, can be applied to the family in Turaba.

Table 10 shows the percentage distribution of the population according to number of family members in the household.

Table - 10
Percent distribution of households according to number of members per household.

Comm.	Households	Number of Members/Household				Total
		1–3	4–6	7–9	>9	
A	87	1	37	47	15	100
B	121	3	42	51	4	100
C	106	3	47	47	3	100

From the table we can see that the large type families (> 9) are very limited, especially among nomads (3 per cent). Several authors such as Patai[62], Leipski[46], describe the Saudi Arabian rural family as an extended one. In our study it is shown that it is more a conjugated rather than an extended family. In Table 11 the total husbands, wives, and children constitute 86 per cent in the settled community and 95 per cent in the nomadic community. It might be that the change from the traditional family to the conjugated family is influenced by the following factors:

1. The migration of the married sons with their families to the cities.

2. The cultivated areas and the number of the livestock are considerably diminished. This, besides the introduction of mechanical devices for agriculture has minimized the need for a large family.

3. With the settlement process, the traditional large nomadic family is broken. On distributing the land in a new settlement area, two small families will have more land than one large family.

Table - 11

**Percent distribution of households according
to relation of members to head.**

Com.	House hold	Total	Head	Wife	Children	Grand Children	Parents	Brothers Sisters	Other Relatives	Total
A	87	551	16	15	55	4	3	2	5	100
B	121	710	17	17	59	2	2	1	2	100
C	161	616	17	16	60	0.3	2	2	2	100

Marriage and Divorce

Marriage: It is unusual for the bridegroom and the bride to see or meet each other before the marriage ceremony. However, in a nomadic community, where there are less restrictions on contact between the two sexes, young couples might meet and talk to each other while watching the flocks or around the camp. Stories about romantic love in Bedouin communities are widely known. Premarital chastity of a woman is an all important social value.

The parents usually choose the bride for their son. A cousin marriage (paternal line) is highly preferable. In some tribes, it is the rule unless the young man does not wish to marry his cousin.

Social and economic factors are always considered in the marriage contract. It is a great stigma for the father if he accepts a husband for his daughter from a tribe of lower status as "Sulaba", from a job of lower status as carpenter, tailor or butcher, or from a race of lower status, as a Negro. All these considerations are, however, less recognized in the heterogeneous community of Souq. The endogenous inbreeding in such isolated communities might have led to the retention of recessive genes.

The bridegroom (or his father) has to pay a bridal payment (Mahar) to the bride's father. Among nomads the payment is in carpets, jewelry, gowns and livestock, rather than in cash. The ceremonies of the marriage parties are a real enjoyment for the people. For three days and nights dancing, music and playing as well as serving of food, are parts of the ceremonies.

A man under the Islamic law has the right to have as many as four wives. "But if You fear that you shall not be able to deal justly (with them), then only one" Qur-an[71]. The prevalence of polygamy in the Islamic countries has been greatly exaggerated in the past by western authors, observers and travelers. "Polygamy has always been, and recently is increasing" (Patai)[63]. In our study the present history of the marital status of the heads of 268 households in the three areas has been taken.* There are ten single, seven divorced, four widowed, and 247 married men. The number of present wives of the married men is shown in Table 12.

Table - 12
Percent distribution of heads of households according to number of their present wives.

Community	Heads	1	2	3	Total
A	59	83	15	2	100
B	107	81	18	1	100
C	81	95	5	0	100

The percentage of polygamy is only 5 percent in the nomad community but 17 to 19 per cent in the settled and semi-settled communities. Lipsky[47] also observed less polygamy among Bedouins than among settled people. In all communities, on average, only one per cent have three wives and none has four wives.

In two studies conducted in four Palestinian villagest[69] and among Sahara tribes[8] the frequency of polygamy varied from 10 to 17 per cent.

---

*   The head is usually the father of the children, but in a few cases he is the elder member of the family.

The main factors appear to determine the extent of polygamy:

1. It is a great burden for a man to have more than one wife. He not only has to pay "Mahar" for the new bride and support two families, but also he has to give his present wife a gift (Ridwaa) which costs almost as much money as the Mahar. Mahar itself becomes a great burden with the competition of the relatively affluent Bedouins working in cities.

2. In a nomadic community it gives social prestige for a man to have more than one wife. However, the father of the bride is usually reluctant to give his daughter to a married man, as she would be forced to share her house with another woman.

Divorce: The man under Islamic law has the right to divorce, but the entire family considerations are likely to determine the frequency of divorce. Divorce among nomads is more simple and more frequent than among the settled communities. There is not much stigma attached to it. The causes of divorce can be mistreatment, barrenness or incompatibility of the temperament of the spouses.

Among nomads, the wife returns to her father's house if her husband beats her. If he beats her three times, by tradition he should divorce her. The woman does not always object to divorce. She can easily get married again (after three monthly periods to be sure she is not pregnant). According to Dickson, "There is no unmarried woman problem, and no prostitution. Adultery or running away with a lover is extremely rare".[13]

The divorced woman usually keeps her children until they are seven years old before she turns them over to the father. Children usually remain in touch with both parents. In the small close community of the Bedouins the divorced husband is still considered as part of the family. Economically the children needs in a Bedouin community are limited, and they are raised among other children in the family.

In a settled community the problem of divorce and its outcome on the children is more complicated. Therefore, divorce is less common.

Child rearing: The child in Turaba enjoys a family with many children around and with inter-family affections and tenderness. Consequently, as the child matures, he is already trained to be a part of a whole and is able to form a group relationship.

Arabia is a man's world[48.] Although marriage confirms the maturity of the individuals involved, only upon the birth of a son are they regarded as full members of the adult community. Among friends and relatives, parents henceforth will ordinarily be addressed as the father or the mother of their first son (using the child's given name). "Women in patriarchal cultures are prouder and more passionate mothers, overly tender to their sons, who largely constitute their own claim to social esteem".[64] There is more joy and celebration upon the birth of a male child.

The child is given his name at the seventh birthday in a big ceremony. Usually two sheep are slaughtered for a male child and one sheep for the female. Although not observed in Turaba, the period of lactation is prolonged to three years for the boy in some tribes.

The difference in the treatment of male and female children (which is more practiced among nomads) is more likely to be reflected in the physical growth of the two sexes in their childhood as well as later on during adulthood.

At the age of two or three years, a male child is circumcised. A big celebration is usually given on this occasion. The operation, conducted by a native practitioner, is usually done under very poor hygienic conditions which may result in infections, adhesions, and deformities. According to Dickson[14,] the American Mission in Kuwait in 1931 used to receive dozens of children whose penises were in a dreadful state of neglect and infection as a result of circumcision. The situation is not far different today. The girls are never circumcised in Turaba. However, the act is said to be practised among other tribes such as Bani Tamim.

Certain ages are considered as milestones in the life of a child. At two years of age, children of both sexes are weaned, and the male child is circumcised.

Until the age of seven years, both boys and girls belong to their mother's world. Besides roaming around with other children, they start to help with the light housework, and the girls are expected to take care of the younger siblings. In that period they are fed the moral codes of the society. The girl is taught to keep her chastity and the boy to become brave and hospitable. Nomads believe that the characteristic traits shaped in early life will never change. "The tail of a dog remains curved, even if it is put into a hundred presses".

The intensity of love which children receive from their parents in early childhood is incredible. "Children are beloved by God". Contrary to what is believed by many authors, corporal punishment of children in a nomadic community is not popular.

At the age of seven years, the boy shifts to his father's world, while the girl becomes more restricted to her mother. The boy starts to enjoy the companionship of his father during the meals in the field and in the men gatherings.

In a nomadic community both boys and girls start herding at the age of seven years, first under the supervision of an older member of the family and then independently at the age of ten to twelve years. In a semi-settled community, whenever a boys' school is available, the boy attends it. "Instruction in childhood is like engraving on a stone". Girls education is still not considered desirable among nomads. The fast progress of girls' education in Souq is a good sign that the negative attitude of Bedouins towards the education of girls will change with time and the availability of schools.

At the age of ten years, girls put on veils, covering the lower half of the face among nomads and semi-nomads, and the whole face in the Souq community. Veiling was not commonly known in the early days of Islam. It was introduced later on as a matter of dignity and to distinguish ladies from slaves. It was further imposed at the time of the Ottoman Empire.

At the age of puberty (14—15 years for both sexes), the person is considered responsible and relatively independent.

MATERNAL AND CHILD HEALTH

MATERNAL HEALTH

Age of Marriage

Among the settled community, girls are married at an average age of 16. Surprisingly, for Bedouin girls it is usually delayed until 18 years of age. A Bedouin girl is needed for herding the goats and sheep. In both communities marriage might be as early as 13 years of age or younger in some cases. It is very unusual to find an unmarried girl at the age of 25 years.

Pregnancy and Abortion

From questioning 352 mothers about the life history of their pregnancy, the average number of pregnancies per mother in the three communities is shown in Table 13.

Table - 13

Average number of pregnancies per mother

Community	Respondents	Average Pregnancies per Mother.
A	100	5.2
B	124	4.9
C	108	5.6

This is however, a selected population of mothers who have children 0––5 years old and have not completed their families. Patai[65] referred to a survey conducted in Palestine in 1945 which shows that the average number of children born by a woman during her lifetime is 9––10.

Knowledge, Attitude & Practice of Family Planning

When we started to ask mothers, "How many children would you like to have?", and "How can a woman prevent the pregnancy?", we faced a great difficulty. The conservative community of Turaba did not accept this type of question. Rumors arose that we were asking about the sexual relationship between the woman and her husband. The female interviewers became more careful in asking the questions, as they had been instructed to avoid the questions if the interviewed woman showed reluctance.

On answering the question, "How many more children do you want to have?", from 14 per cent in Souq to 29 per cent in semi-settled community said that they wanted more children (Table 14). I believe that this is an underestimate, since most of the interviewed mothers are young and are shy in expressing their desire for more children.

Table - 14

Response of mothers to the question of how many more children they want to have.

Com.	Resp.	No more	More	As God Wished	Wants Health	Other	Does not know
A	80	21	14	29	13	2	1
B	99	20	29	31	14	4	1
C	85	19	18	22	16	4	6

About 50 per cent in all communities responded to the question by either saying "as God wishes" or "I want health". This was matter of shyness, fatalism, or to avoid the evil eye.

One mother said, "I want as many children as the papers in your hand". Another one wanted five boys and one girl. "The boys will take care of me, and the girl will take care of her husband".

An Aramco survey in the Eastern province showed that six children is the desired number among villagers. Males were preferred[21]. In the 1930's Dickson said, "Every Arabian woman's greatest desire in life is to have a child, . . . she will be divorced if she will not produce a son and heir for her husband".[15]

Children are wanted as a source of support, comfort in old age, power against enemies, and after death, help into heaven.

Contraception

The mother, if she were cooperative, was asked if a woman can prevent pregnancy and how (Table 15).

Table - 15

Percent distribution of mothers responding to the question "Can a woman prevent pregnancy?"

Com.	No.	Yes	No	Don't Know	Total
A	79	32	14	54	100
B	94	3	10	87	100
C	73	--	7	93	100

Thirty-two per cent in Souq said that prevention of pregnancies is possible, against 3 per cent in semi-settled and none in nomadic communities. The majority said that they didn't know. This is either due to ignorance or shyness. All those who said contraception was possible mentioned pills as the means of contraception except two who mentioned injections. Apparently many of those who mentioned pills might have never seen them.

My impression is that contraceptions are used sometimes, particularly if a woman has enough children (especially boys). Pills are known on a small scale in Souq, otherwise local herbs are used.

Abortion

In the last year there were eight abortions among the interviewees in the three communities (2.5 per cent).

A woman is thought to have an abortion if she lifts a heavy weight, is beaten by per husband, or is affected by a supernatural power (God, Jinn, Evil Eye). (Jinn cause abortion as well as sterility, death of the children, or delay of childbirth for several years).

We did not dare to ask about induced abortion even in an informal way. The only old Bedouin lady whom we asked about it got very angry, and her enraged reply was, "It is for prostitutes". Although induced abortion might be practiced occasionally, the religious feeling against it is very strong.

Sterility

The woman is usually thought to be responsible for the unproductivity. A man, however, is considered responsible in rare cases. The causes of man's sterility are (1) smallpox, (2) Jin. The causes of woman's sterility are (1) sickness, (2) deformity or blockage of the womb, (3) a Jin takes the spermatozoa away, (4) the woman herself stepping over a grave.

Treatment of sterility in women includes (1) Saiid –– to treat Al Jinni, (2) "Thuffa" is left in a bottle of water for overnight under the stars, to be drunk the next morning, (3) the woman sits over a utensil filled with water and drops seven hot small stones in the water. Apparently, failure to cure an obscure and mysterious condition like sterility with herbs and cautery leads to the usage of supernatural methods.

Antenatal Care

The mothers were asked about their present pregnancy (Table 16).

Table - 16
Percent distribution of pregnant women interviewed

Comm.	Number	Pregnant Mothers	%
A	100	21	21
B	124	20	17
C	108	22	20

Of those, only five pregnant mothers from Community A and three pregnant mothers from Communities B and C sought medical care in the health center during the period of the pregnancy for partum or related conditions (e.g. haemorrhage, discharge, abdominal pain, etc.). The doctor in the Health Center never examined a patient vaginally. He usually refers a case of, say, haemorrhage to the female nurse. The ultimate advice to the patient, whether she accepts the examination or not, is to go to Taif. This action is rarely taken because of the long distance from Taif, ignorance and fatalism.

Natal and Postnatal care

In all communities, there is no Daia (local midwife) system which exists in other areas of the country. All deliveries are assisted by female relatives or neighbors. In the last year, however, the female nurse has attended seven deliveries out of 47 total deliveries in Souq. Basically, in all communities there is no objection from man or women to the nurse attending the delivery. Even the male doctor may attend if it is necessary

A lady in Souq told me that she does not mind, and even wants the nurse to attend her delivery. However, she is afraid that she cannot "honor" the nurse by giving her enough money (although she is not obligated). This is similar to what the Jordanian agricultural engineer told me. "The people want us to help them, but they are reluctant to call upon us. This is mostly because they cannot afford to slaughter a sheep for us, which is a shameful thing not to do".

The expenses of the transportation of the nurse or the doctor to the villages and nomadic areas add to the problem.

All the 136 deliveries which had occurred last year in all three communities have been attended at home except one delivery from Community B which was attended in Taif.

No special preparation for delivery is made. The basic rule is that no one should interfere with the delivery. The delivering mother pulls on a rope attached to the roof and a woman braces her from behind. The other women wait patiently.

After birth, the umbilical cord is cut by a knife or a scissor, and then the tool is washed carefully from the blood (ritual) and put under the child's pillow to protect him from Jinn. The baby is washed with water (soap hurts him), kohl is put in his eyes, and he is given a lick of samna (ghee) to lubricate his intestines and clean out the dirt. The child is then wrapped in tight clothes and kept away from the eyes of strangers (to avoid Evil Eye).

The mother cleans herself with warm water. Her food would consist of Asida (wheat and ghee) honey and meat. The food will be enriched by "hot" herbs (pepper, thuffa and helba). The mother usually stays in bed for 7––14 days, but never does any hard work before 40 days. Her neighbours bring her food and take care of her house.

In cases of complication little can be done. "God will save her or she dies". Bleeding is beyond their control. In case she faints, they put cooled "boiled oil" on her head. The settled people claim that a Bedouin woman still uses a vaginal pack of common salt "to reduce the size".

Basically the difference between Souq and the other two communities is a difference in the environmental condition (housing and availability of water) rather than a difference in health knowledge or attitude.

NUTRITION

" **P**eople like what they eat, rather than eat what they like". Kurt Lewin[45].

The female interviewers interviewed the mothers in Turaba about nutrition of the family as a whole and of the children in particular. Informal open-ended questions were held to learn more about the cultural values of foods and the customs related to them.

We faced some difficulties in this part of the study. For instance, in estimating the quantity of rice eaten "yesterday", the mother would demonstrate the quantity either by her hand or by a local home utensil. The interviewer would convert the demonstrated amount into a standardized local measurement "Robaa" (800 gm.) and then to a metric measurement. In estimating the quantities consumed per month, we depended on the memory of the respondent. A nutritional survey based on a day by day estimation was beyond our ability. The problems of recall, human error of the interviewers, the motivation of the respondents, as well as other problems of reliability and validity of assessment have been faced in many nutritional studies[81,26].

FAMILY NUTRITION

We asked the mothers about the family consumption of certain types of food in two periods, "yesterday" and during the last month. The average number of household members participating in the last evening meal was 3.1 adults and

3.4 children, with no difference between the communities. No attempt was made, however, to adjust for the age of children which may go up to 15 years.

Table 17 shows the percentage of families who mentioned eating specific types of food "yesterday".

Table - 17
Percent of households who mentioned eating specific types of food "yesterday".

Com.	Resp.	Meat	Vegetables	Fruit	Milk	Date	Tea	Coffee
A	77	68	53	16	36	62	51	98
B	117	6	4	—	18	82	78	93
C	80	8	1	—	16	86	78	86

Apparently, families in Souq consumed more meat, vegetables, fruit and milk than families in the other two communities. More people in the semi-settled and the nomadic communities reported that they had consumed dates, tea and coffee.

This table is probably a good reflection of the difference of the nutritional status of the three communities.

People in Souq consume more varieties of foods including meat, vegetables and fruits, while the semi-settled and nomadic communities depend largely on flour, rice, dates and tomato paste with little and occasional variations.

Meat

Fourty-four per cent in Souq consumed ½ kg. meat per day and 23 per cent consumed more than that. In the last month, more than half of the people in Souq consumed 5 kg. per month. In the semi-settled and the nomadic communities the main occasion for eating meat is when someone is invited to their homes or if they get invited out. In the previous month 62 per cent and

77 per cent from Communities B and C, respectively, had eaten meat when a sheep was slaughtered for a guest, either by their family or by their neighbors.

Thirty-four per cent in semi-settled community and 19 per cent in the nomadic community have bought meat from a butcher in the last month. This is a new trend occurring recently with the severity of the drought and the diminishing quantities of animals. A man buys his supply of meat when he goes to Souq or Alawa market for the Friday Prayer. Interestingly, the four butchers in the two markets are either Yemenis or Negroes. They are never from the Bedouin tribes, who put a stigma on this type of work.

Rice

Only 9 respondents in all communities said they did not eat rice yesterday. Rice along with bread is the most staple food, particularly in the semi-settled and nomadic communities. There is no apparent difference in the amount of rice consumed per day by the three communities.

Flour

It was difficult to compare the amount of flour consumed per family per day in the three communities. In Souq, most of the people buy bread loves from the market, whereas in the other two communities, people make their own bread at home. In all communities, only one respondent in Community B mentioned that the family did not eat bread "yesterday".

Vegetables

The frequency of vegetable consumption –– molloukhia, bamia (okra), dubba (pumpkins), koosa (zucchini), basal (onion) and badinjan (tomato) per family per month in the three communities was studied. Whereas 52 per cent in Community A consumed vegetables more than four times per month, only

3 per cent and 2 per cent in Communities B and C, respectively, consumed that amount per month. Nine per cent and 8 per cent in Communities B and C, respectively, said that they eat vegetables occasionally. The main single occasion is when relatives working in the cities pay a short visit or spend the summer vacation with their families in Turaba. They then bring with them varieties of vegetables, fruits, seeds, cereals and nuts.

Although vegetables as well as fruits are readily available in the markets of Souq and Alawa, the Bedouins are not interested in buying them. They either do not like them, do not know how to cook them, or cannot afford them. What is more important, they do not attach any nutritional value to them as they do to meat.

Eggs

Eggs are not a common dish among people even in Souq. Thirty-two per cent in Souq, 4 per cent in the semi-settled community and 2 per cent in the nomadic community reported that they ate eggs in the last month. Many semi-settled and nomadic people said, "Eggs! We have never tasted them".

Raising chickens does not fit in with the wandering life of the nomadic Bedouins. Now, even after some of them have settled, chickens do not have the social value of goats and sheep. No Bedouin can provide his guest with chicken.

Milk

Milk is the most preferred food after meat. However, it is not always available. One of the Bedouins said to me, "We never knew these diseases when we use to eat meat and drink milk". Goat's milk, if available, is the favorite, and the next best is sheep's milk. Camel's milk is a "strong" milk, and for those who are not accustomed to it, it causes diarrhea. Powdered milk has a much lower status than fresh milk.

Butter

When fresh milk is lacking, animal butter is also rather scarce. People in Turaba use canned vegetable samna (ghee). It is an essential part of their cooking when it is available. Many of the old people attribute their rheumatic pains and weakness to the canned samna, "which is doubtless made of vaseline". However, they still use it because it is better than nothing.

Dates

The date is one of the most important foods among nomads and the semi-settled. It is eaten with practically every meal and between meals. It is also served with coffee and tea at social gatherings and during visits.

In summary, the daily basic food for the people in the three communities is:

1. Breakfast: bread, dates, tea and coffee.

2. Lunch: rice and tomato sauce made of tomato paste, onion and samna (ghee) or Margoog made of small balls of bread soaked in tomato sauce.

3. Dinner: bread and tomato sauce or margoog.

In Souq, occasionally meat, vegetables and fruits are added to lunch or dinner, and sometimes powdered milk to breakfast. Nomads and semi-settled consume meat less frequently and mainly when a guest is invited either by the household at home or by the neighbors. Less variations of food exist in the latter two communities.

CHILD NUTRITION

Of our respondents, 65 per cent in Souq, 94 per cent of the semi-settled and 92 per cent of the nomads said that they give their children samna (ghee) at birth for the first three days of life. "It lubricates the intestine, cleans it, and gives the child nourishment". In case samna is not available, drops of castor oil are given to the baby, and a lactating neighbor or relative is called to breast feed the baby until his mother lactates in the second or third day. In that case, the wet nurse is considered by religious beliefs as the child's second mother and there would be no intermarriage between the two women's children. Some of the nomadic Bedouins extend the samna-licking until the seventh day after birth, and in exceptional cases until the fortieth day.

Table 18 shows the type of milk fed to the children in the three communities by age group.

Table - 18
Type of milk feeding of children under the study by age group.

Com.	Age Group	No.	Breast	Powdered	Goat	Weaned
	−1	33	17	11	2	3
	−2	26	12	8	1	5
A	2+	104	−	2	1	101
	all ages	163	32	18	4	109
	−1	39	35	1	1	2
	− 2	37	26	6	1	4
B	2+	118	3	−	−	115
	all ages	194	62	7	2	121
	−1	29	27	1	−	1
−	2	29	22	1	1	5
C	2 +	102	−	2	−	100
	all ages	160	49	4	1	106

Breast feeding is the predominant method of feeding for children up to two years of age in the three communities. Feeding with powdered milk is one of the main differences in the nutrition of children between the three communities. While 19 (32 per cent) of children <2 years old in Souq are given powdered milk, only 7 (9 per cent) and 2 (4 per cent) of the same age group in semi-settled and nomadic communities, respectively, are given powdered milk. In Souq powdered milk is considered as a sign of modernization.

In semi-settled and nomadic communities powdered milk is used occasionally if the mother is sick or if the child is unable to suck her breast. A wet nurse, either hired or volunteered, is far more preferable to powdered milk. This is not only because powdered milk is expensive, but also because human milk is highly preferable to any other kind of milk. An Arabic proverb says, "Character impressed by the mother's milk cannot be altered by anything except death".

Goat's milk, if available, is given to grown children but rarely to young children, since it causes "Tukhma" (anorexia and diarrhea). Breast feeding is practiced in the easy-going self-demand method, a method which is also recommended by some modern authorities. The duty of the mother is to quiet the child with her breast milk and never let him cry for a prolonged period of time; otherwise he will get Bakwa (epileptic fit).

Among the people I asked, I did not find discrimination against female babies in breast feeding. Discrimination does exist however in solid food feeding. One of the female interviewers reported that some Bedouin mothers give their male children the breast for more than 24 months, a longer period than for females. This preference for males over females has been found by Puyet[70] among Arab refugees in Lebanon.

Solid Food

Table 19 shows the age at which semi-solids and solid foods are introduced to children.

Table - 19
Percent distribution of age of introducing solid foods to babies

Community	No.	6	6--9	10--12	>12	Total
			Age in Months			
A	97	10	54	29	7	100
B	121	23	42	31	4	100
C	101	17	44	33	6	100

Mostly, the introduction of solid food commences at the age of 6 to 9 months. At that age the child is given Al Easha, (piece of bread, rice or date) to suck on. Then gradually the child is given what is available on the food table and at any time in the day. Meat is not given at this time as it is "too heavy" for very young children. A child is allowed to suck meat when he is around one and a half years old, but is not allowed to eat it before the age of two years.

A change has occurred in the last year in Souq, where a child might be given canned preserved food if it can be afforded.

Weaning

The vast majority of mothers (>90 per cent) in all communities wean their children at exactly two years of age or earlier if they become pregnant. Weaning here means the completion of the weaning process when the child is prevented from breast feeding. The milk of a pregnant mother is thought to be toxic for her child. It might affect him by Ghoosh (diarrhea and bulging abdomen). In Souq it appears that weaning before two years (for reasons other than pregnancy) is practiced more than the other two communities. It is strongly believed that a child must be weaned in the same week or even on the day of becoming two years of age. People believe that this is ordered by God. It has been recommended by the Quran and by the prophet Mohammed that a child better be weaned at this age[60], but it is never mandatory[72]. Jalliffe4 1 mention the same belief among people in Lebanon, Syria, Iraq and Morocco.

Buck in his study in Chad found that 92 per cent of the mothers in Djimtito, a predominant Muslim community, wean their children at two years of age.

Weaning is done abruptly. Various methods are used in different areas to distract the child from the breast. The most common one is to put myrrh or black pepper on the breast of the mother. Among Bedouins another method still commonly used is to prick the nose of the child with a pin every time he approaches the breast. A less commonly used method is to apply drops of a small insect's blood on the breast.

Preschool Children

After weaning, the two year old child is allowed to eat every kind of food available, including meat. At the age of three years the child sits regularly at three meals with the members of the family except the father, who in nomadic and semi-nomadic communities usually eats the noon and evening meals with his neighbors, friends or guests.

At the age of five to seven years the male child is allowed to join his father except in the presence of strangers. A male child is always highly favored with the best food. "A male child is a much valued arrival in the family, to him is passed the honor of the family, and upon him rests the responsibility of maintaining it". Lipsky[48].

NUTRITIONAL IMPACT ON THE HEALTH OF THE CHILDREN

From the previous presentation it is apparent that there is a difference in the quantity and quality of food consumption in the settled and nomadic communities. People in Souq, mainly for economic considerations consume more animal protein (meat, milk and eggs), vegetables and fruit than the other two communities.

The possible effect of the difference in the nutritional status of settled and nomadic communities will be discussed in relation to three phases of child development —— pre-weaning, weaning and post weaning periods.

Pre-Weaning Period. In the first six months the majority of children in all communities are breast fed. At that stage the mother's milk is relatively adequate quantitatively and qualitatively for the development of the child. The child's growth is, however, affected by the nutrition of his mother. Suckling anemia and infantile beri beri are common findings among infants born to anemic mothers or mothers with deficiency of thiamin in rice-eating communities[85]. This condition is likely to be more prevalent in the semi-settled and nomadic communities. However, with the trend of artificial feeding started recently in Souq, infants are more apt to have diarrhea.

Weaning period. This period starts in all communities at the age of six to nine months when solid and semi-solid foods are introduced. It continues until two years, the age of weaning completion. This is the most critical period of a child's life. The child faces a sudden change to adult type of food which is poor hygienically and less nutritious. The nomad and the semi-settled children are more likely to be subjected to the synergetic action of malnutrition and infectious diseases.

The mother's milk is insufficient both quantitatively and qualitatively in that period. Solid food, high in carbohydrate and low in protein and vitamin values gives insufficient needs for a growing child. This is especially so in the nomadic community.

According to Gordon[28], the majority of deaths of children in underdeveloped countries occur in the weaning period. The peak of deaths from diarrhea in his study in rural India occurred around the tenth month of life. The hypothesis is that in a malnourished individual, organisms not normally pathogenic may cause diarrheal disease or contribute to its development.

Post-weaning period. In Guatemala the introduction of a nutritional program for pre-school children in a village improved the mortality rate4. Still, it is a critical period of the child's life. The child in a nomadic community continues to eat from the available household food, with high carbohydrate and less protein. The young children eat with their mothers and young siblings from less nutritious food than their fathers. The previously consumed mother's milk (although insufficient) was better than the solid food.

The growth curves (Figure 4 and 5) show that the weight of children, particularly females in the nomadic community, depart increasingly from the Harvard standard growth curve. The traditional preference for male children over female children among Bedouins showed in the relatively higher growth curves for males.

SANITARY ENVIRONMENT

Housing:

Construction

Houses in Souq are built from mud or bricks. They are big and roomy compared to the mud houses and beehive huts in Hejar. Bedouins live in their traditional black tents made from goat's hair. The surface area of a tent may vary in size from 20–40 square meters. It is usually divided into three compartments for cooking, living and sleeping. None of the three types of dwelling is insect or rodent proof.

Occupancy

There is no significant difference between the average number of persons living in a household in the three communities. It ranges from 6.3 in Community A to 5.7 in Community C. However, concerning the size and the type of the houses in the three communities, the level of crowding is higher in the nomadic community, moderate in the semi-settled community and lower in Souq.

Cleanliness

In general, houses in the three communities are moderately clean. However, the courtyards and areas surrounding mud houses, particularly in Souq, are in many cases filled by garbage. A Bedouin tent is generally less clean than a mud house in Souq, but the surrounding area is, no doubt, cleaner. In the summer when a large group of Bedouins camp around a dug well, the group moves gradually in an outward direction whenever the camp area becomes filled with the manure of the animals.

Ventilation

Ventilation in tents is excellent. In Souq and Hejar mud and hut houses it is less than adequate.

Water:

Shallow to deep dug wells (10—–20 meters deep) are the source of water in all communities. In the nomadic communities water is drawn from the well by a can attached to a rope, and carried to homes by water-skin.

In the agricultural communities (A and B), most of the wells are provided with pumps. Water is pumped from the well to a small pool about one meter above the surface of the ground, where it is used for agricultural and domestic purposes.

In Souq water is carried to homes by a man (sagga) or by drums driven by donkeys. Only for the Development Center and the school is the water carried by truck. A few houses are provided with small water tanks; otherwise water is kept in large water jars.

Samples of water were taken in sterilized bottles from seven wells in different communities and from household utensils in Ergain. The water samples were shipped by plane from Jeddah to the central laboratory in Riyadh. Because the specimens were delayed about ten days during shipment, only chemical examination was possible. The results of the examination are, as follows:

Test	Range of findings in all samples
NO_2	nil-traces
NO_3	nil
Ca	60––80 mg./liter
Ma	17––32 mg./liter
Fe	traces
Mn	nil
Cl	109––600 mg./liter
$CaCo_3$	210––730 mg./liter
Soluble Salts	480––780 mg./liter
P.H.	7.5 –– 7.8

All the above findings are considered normal by the WHO International Standards for Drinking Water[92].

However, ammonia, a probable sign of pollution was detected in three samples which were drawn from a shallow well in Kara, a pool used as a water reservoir in Souq and a household utensil in Ergain (.04, .08, 0.6 mg./liter).

Water in all communities, particularly the nomadic community, is highly subjected to contamination from the time it is in the shallow unprotected wells, through the process of transportation and storage, until the time of usage.

Excreta Disposal:

Based on questionnaires, the presence of latrines in the three communities is shown in Table 20.

Table - 20

Distribution of households provided with latrines.

| | | Latrines Present | |
Community	Number of Household	Number	Per cent
A	60	43	72
B	106	2	2
C	86	0	0

The latrines in Souq are of cesspool or pit privy types. They are inadequately protected, and the surrounding area is not always clean.

In the semi-settled and the nomadic communities the distance of the defecation site from the house varies from 20—50 meters (shorter for females). Cleaning is done by water, if available; otherwise by graves. The defecation sites in nomadic areas are dry and unshady, while in agricultural communities they are generally shady and moist. It is more likely that the stool disposal act in a settled or semi-settled areas, either in the latrine or around the house, is more hazardous than it is in the desert.

Food Sanitation:

Undercooked food and food kept overnight are thought to cause diarrhea. Whenever it is possible, food is consumed the same day. Food is a "blessing" and throwing it away is undesirable. Extra food, however, is thrown to animals or simply in the back yards in Souq. Milk is always boiled, since unboiled milk is thought to cause diarrhea and abdominal pains.

Fortunately, bottled-feeding practice is not yet common, particularly among nomads. The few demonstrations we saw for the preparation of bottles were terribly unsanitary. The bottle was usually rinsed in cold water. If powdered milk was used, half the required amount was added. The nipple was manipulated frequently, and more than one child might use the bottle.

Personal Hygiene:

Cleanness is a basic concept in Islam. "Wash your garments, shorten your hair, use toothpicks, adorn yourselves and keep clean".[57] Most of these recommendations are practiced whenever it is possible, especially before the Friday prayer. However, scarcity of water and ignorance determine the capability of people, particularly nomads, to keep the recommendations.

Regarding our question, "What are the advantages of settlement over nomadism?", cleanness was mentioned by 79 per cent of settled people in Souq and 31 per cent of nomadic Bedouins.

Insects and Rodents:

Table 21 indicates flies were the most complained of insects in the three communities. Roaches were mentioned almost exclusively in Souq where latrines and water drainage are built into houses. Mosquitoes, rats, scorpions and snakes are more of a problem for the semi-settled and nomadic communities where houses are less protected from field pests than in Souq.

Table - 21
Percent distribution of the most commonly mentioned pests and insects.

Community	Households	Mosquitoes	Flies	Roaches	Rats	Scorpions and Snakes
A	34	29	85	52	11	35
B	46	69	89	4	84	86
C	33	51	87	–	81	66

HEALTH STATUS

CHILDREN

Morbidity

Mothers were interviewed by the female interviewers about the health conditions of their children. They were asked about the presence of four selected complaints: diarrhea, cough, fever and eye disease.

Diarrhea. Diarrhea is defined as five or more loose stools/day in the case of infants below one year and three or more stools/day in the case of children of two to four years. An attempt was made at the beginning of the study to inquire about additional signs and symptoms accompanied with diarrhea such as character of stool and presence of blood in cases of children of two to four years, in order to grade the severity of diarrhea. However, in most instances, especially in nomadic and semi-nomadic areas, we found that the mother was not aware of the character of the stool since the older children defecate in the field or the surrounding areas.

Table 22 shows the prevalence of the four selected complaints among children in the three communities by age group.

Essentially there is no difference in distribution of age groups in the three communities. There is a consistently lower rate of complaints in Souq than in semi-settled and nomadic communities except in diarrhea among

0‒‒11 months age group. The difference between semi-settled and nomadic communities is not consistent. While the semi-settled group has lower rates than the nomadic in eye diseases and diarrhea, it has a higher rate of cough and fever. The high prevalence of cough in the nomadic group and more particularly in the semi-settled, can be attributed to the epidemic wave of whooping cough at the time of the study.

Table - 22
Percent distribution of children 0‒‒5 years with four selected complaints.

Age in months	Community	Number of Children	Diarrhea	Cough	Fever	Eye Disease
	A	33	9	18	9	12
0‒‒11	B	39	8	49	18	28
	C	29	17	34	21	45
	A	26	12	8	15	8
12‒‒23	B	37	32	35	22	16
	C	29	24	45	24	34
	A	104	8	14	10	8
24‒‒59	B	118	11	41	19	23
	C	102	14	38	12	29
	A	163	9	13	10	9
All ages	B	194	14	41	19	23
	C	160	16	39	16	33

Diarrhea prevalence in the three communities shows its peak among the age group of 1‒‒2 years. Its prevalence among this age group is significantly different from the other two age groups (‒‒ 1 yr, 2 + yrs) (p =<0.005).

Table 23 shows the two-week period prevalence of the same four complaints among children. Souq has lower prevalence than the other two communities in all conditions except diarrhea.

Table - 23
Percent distribution of children 0––5 years with 2 week history of four selected complaints.

Community	Number of Children	Diarrhea	Cough	Fever	Eye Disease
A	163	22	17	17	12
B	194	24	41	28	31
C	160	19	40	26	29

In summary we can say that there was no difference between the children in the three communities in the incidence of diarrhea. Cough and eye disease both were significantly higher in nomadic and semi-settled communities. Fever was also higher in the latter two communities, but was only of borderline significance.

Accidents:

Table 24 shows the percentage of children reported to have selected accidents during the last year. All accidents were reported among children above one year of age in semi-settled and nomads, and above two years of age in Souq. The highest incidence of kerosene drinking and burns was among children 1––2 years old in semi-settled and nomads and 2––4 years old in Souq. All animal bites (dogs) and venom bites (snakes and scorpions) in semi settled and nomads were reported among children 2––4 years old, while none of these two types of accidents was reported in Souq.

Table - 24
Percent distribution of children who had accidents
during the preceeding year.

Community	No.	Burns	Kerosene Drinking	Venom Bites	Animal
A	163	4	4	––	––
B	194	5	3	1	4
C	160	4	2	1	3

Infant Mortality Rate (IMR)

Table 25 shows the preceding years live births, number of deaths among 0––1 year old children, and the calculated infant mortality rate.

The apparent difference between the three communities in the IMR was not statistically significant at the 5% level as the sample size was not large enough to detect such a difference.

Some years ago, Dickson[16] observed that among 15 Bedouin children perhaps only three or four survive.

Table - 25
Live births, infant deaths and infant mortality rate
in the preceding year.

Community	No. of Mothers	Live Births	Infant Deaths	IMR/1000
A	100	47	4	85
B	124	48	8	166
C	108	39	7	179
Total	332	134	19	134

My personal impression is that these figures are not sufficiently reliable, since our cross sectional study depended a great deal on the memory of the mother. Any future studies on IMR should be based on longitudinal surveys and births and deaths registers.

ADULTS

The heads of the households and the mothers of children were asked about the history of their morbidity during the last two weeks (Tables 26 and 27).

Table - 26
Percent distribution of heads of households with history of morbidity in the preceding two weeks.

Com.	No.	No Complaint	Body Aches	Chest & Abdominal Pains	Weakness	Eye Dis.	Other Specific	Other Non-Specific
A	61	52	28	8	2	5	2	15
B	108	41	37	18	7	3	2	10
Could	89	50	28	8	2	1	1	18

Table - 27

Percent distribution of mothers with history of morbidity in the preceding two weeks.

Com.	No.	No Complaint	Body Aches	Chest & Abdominal Pains	Weakness	Cough	Other Specific	Other Non-Specific
A	98	57	21	7	5	2	1	12
B	124	20	51	23	4	6	2	13
C	103	14	50	14	11	7	1	22

Body aches and headaches were the most frequently reported complaints among males and females in all communities. Chest and abdominal pains came in the next place. Both of these conditions were reported more among females in semi-settled and nomadic communities than in Souq. In all communities, weakness was a common complaint among males and females. While more males mentioned eye complaints, more females complained of cough. Diarrhea was rarely mentioned, probably because of an attached stigma in the local culture. A peculiar feature is that no more than 2% of the whole population complained of specific diseases. This was unexpected at least in Souq where people have better education and more accessibility to health centers in Turaba and Taif.

RESULT OF CLINICAL EXAMINATION, ANTHROPOMETRIC MEASUREMENTS AND LABORATORY TESTS.

Clinical Examination

Selected clinical signs were chosen as indicators for nutritional and infectious diseases. Table 29 shows the prevalence of these selected conditions among the children 0—5 years old. There is no apparent difference in the prevalence of the conditions between the three communities except in ulcers ($p = <$ 0.01) and infected penis ($p = <$ 0.005), also no obvious difference between males and females in any of the three communities except in pediculosis and conjunctivitis which are always higher among females.

Table - 28
Percent distribution of positive clinical findings among children 0––5 years.

Community	A	B	C
Respondents	101	133	98

Clinical Findings

	A	B	C
Hair depigmentation	2	2	4
Nasolabial seborrhea	2	1	1
Angular stomatitis	3	2	3
Acute conjunctivitis	12	14	19
Ulcers	2	11	8
Infected penis	––	8	7
Pediculosis	21	15	21
Liver enlargement	4	4	3
Spleen enlargement	––	––	––
Leg edema	2	8	5
Marasmus	2	4	3

Malnutrition: The prevalence of the clinical signs of malnutrition as hair depigmentation, nasolabial seborrhea and angular stomatitis is not significantly different in the three communities ($p = < 0.30$).

There were a total of 21 children with one or more positive clinical signs of malnutrition (hair depigmentation, nasolabial seborrhea, angular stomatitis and leg edema). Out of these, there were five cases who had more than one important clinical sign of kwashiorkor. There were no indications of any linkage of malnutrition with the sex of the child.

Due to the small number of observed conditions, no definite correlation between the prevalence of the condition and the age of the children could be determined except in a few cases. In all communities, no sign of nutritional deficiency was observed in children under one year of age. The same is true of pediculosis. Conjunctivitis has relatively high prevalence among children below one year of age –– 33% of all cases in Souq, 49% in semi-settled and 42% in the nomadic community. Small-pox scars were found in 35 children in Souq, 21 children in semi-settled and 9 children in the nomadic community.

The lack of difference between the three communities in the prevalence of the clinical signs of malnutrition does not reflect the anthropometric findings which will be discussed later, for it shows a significant difference between Souq and the nomadic community.

Other nutritional studies indicate that the clinical findings, being insensitive, do not always reflect the nutritional status of a population[38, 39]. Although some typical cases of kwashiorkor have been seen in this study, sub-clinical cases might exist undiagnosed[91]. Infantile beri beri, an expected condition in communities B and C which depends largely on polished rice as the main staple food, might have already led to some infantile deaths.

In a nutritional assessment study conducted in Jordan among refugee children 0––4 years old[36] an almost similar prevalence of signs of malnutrition was found among the studied population (7% hair depigmentation, 2.5% angular lesions, 4.5% marasmus and 1% kwashiorkor). In that study, there was no correlation between the clinical findings and the sex.

Conjunctivitis is less prevalent in this dry part of the country than in the Eastern Province where trachoma effects 90% of the school age children and older[56]. Conjunctival scarring as entropion and ectropion was not revealed. However, the absence of gross scarification does not exclude the possibility of the existence of trachoma in a community[32].

Taylor[83], in his study of conjunctivitis in the Punjab, related the widespread nature of conjunctivitis among young children to the local habit of applying black paste, "kohl", by a small stick to the eyes of the members of the family. This habit which is still prevalent, particularly among the Bedouins, might be of some importance in the prevalence of the condition. Other factors, such as the low hygienic conditions, overcrowding and the prevalence of house flies, might play a role in the prevalence of the condition.

Ulcers and Infected Penis: Ulcers observed are either traumatic or the result of infected cautery. Infected penis in all observed cases was the result of unhygienic process of circumcising of young male children.

Although cautery and circumcision are practiced at homes in all communities, the observed favorable outcome of both procedures in Souq might be due to more sterile techniques, better post-operative hygiene or the availability of antibacterial drugs in the Health Center.

Anthropometric Measurements

The manner in which height, weight, head circumference and chest circumference change with age in months was determined according to least squares polynomial equation[19.] The form of each equation is:

$$Y^1 = b_0 \qquad b_1 A - b_2 A^2$$

where A = age in months

b_0, b_1, b_2 = least squares partial
regression coefficient

The predicted height and weight for males and females in the three communities by age group are shown in Table 29.

Table - 29
Predicted Height and Weight for Males and Females in the Three Communities by Age Group (in months)

Measurement	Com	3 Male	3 Female	6 Male	6 Female	12 Male	12 Female	24 Male	24 Female	36 Male	36 Female	48 Male	48 Female	60 Male	60 Female
Height in cm	A	61.3	59.0	64.4	62.6	70.0	69.2	79.7	80.2	87.0	88.4	92.0	93.7	94.7	96.???
	B	59.4	59.6	61.6	62.1	66.1	66.9	74.8	75.8	83.2	83.8	91.3	90.0	96.1	95.???
	C	57.5	56.0	61.0	59.0	67.5	66.3	78.3	75.5	86.2	83.4	91.2	89.0	93.4	92.???
Weight in kg	A	5.8	5.1	6.5	5.9	7.8	7.3	9.9	9.8	11.5	11.6	12.5	12.7	12.9	13.???
	B	5.5	5.2	6.0	5.7	7.0	6.7	8.9	8.5	10.7	10.1	12.3	11.5	13.4	12.???
	C	4.9	4.3	5.6	4.9	6.9	6.0	9.2	8.1	10.8	9.8	11.9	11.2	12.4	12.???

There is a significant difference between the children in the three communities in weight and height. The differences are largely between females rather than males and especially observed in the nomadic community. This difference in the measurements of the two sexes in the nomadic community might be due to the preference for males over females. The same difference between male and female measurements was found by other workers, as Neumann in her Punjab study[59] and Morley in West Africa[54].

For the sake of clarity, the heights and weights of children in the two main populations, settled and nomadic are plotted in Figures 4 and 5. Harvard standard[58] measurements (50th percentile) were selected as standards of reference and plotted against Turaba growth curves.

In figure 4 the weight and height of male children of Souq and the nomadic community are plotted against the Harvard standard for male children. For both measurements the local curves start at almost the same level as the Harvard curve, and then increasingly depart from the latter. Also, for both measurements, the Souq curve is above that for the nomadic community and nearly parallel to it. However, the difference was not proven to be statistically significant.

In figure 5 the weight and height of female children in Souq and the nomadic community were plotted against the Harvard standards. Here again, the local curves start approximately at the same level as the Harvard curve and then depart widely, particularly in weight. The female differences in both height and weight were proven to be statistically significant. The differences are more striking in weight than in height.

A similar deviation from Boston Standard was observed by Taha[82] among Sudanese children, sexes combined.

Normally, the chest to head ratio exceeds 1 after six months of age[42.] In our population this predicted ratio exceeds 1 among males only at the age of three years, whereas among females it remains below 1 even at that age. This might indicate a low nutritional status and hindrance to normal growth, especially among females.

The retardation in the children's growth relative to the Harvard statistics might be explained by hereditary factors as well as the effect of the synergetic action between malnutrition and infectious diseases. The difference in the growth of male and female children in the nomadic community might be explained by the observed cultural difference in the treatment of the two sexes. In the settled community the girls as well as the boys enjoy relatively better nourishment than in the Bedouin community.

Laboratory Investigations

Haemoglobin: Table 30 shows the percentage distribution of the haemoglobin value in gm % among the studied group of children 0—5 years in the three communities. The children in Souq have a higher percentage of readings above 10 gm%. If a haemoglobin value of less than 10 gm% is taken as an indication of anaemia[40], this would indicate a higher prevalence of anaemia among young children in semi-settled and nomadic communities.

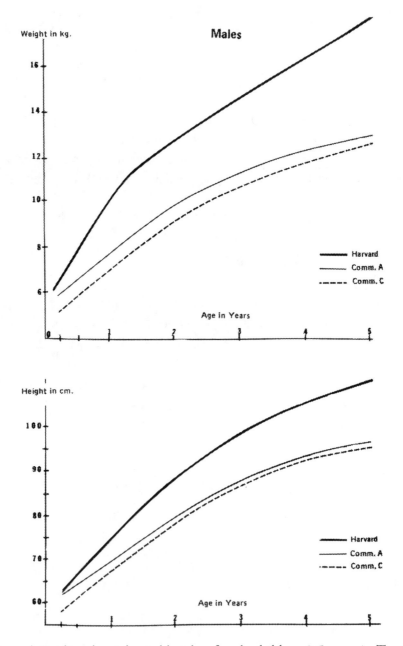

Figure 4. Predicted weight and height of male children 0-5 years in Turaba (communities A,C) compared to Harvard standard (50th percentile).

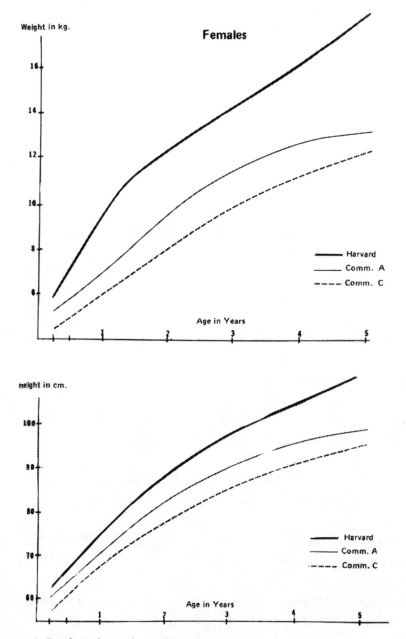

Figure 5. Predicted weight and height of female children 0-5 years in Turaba (communities A,C) compared to Harvard standard (50th percentile).

Zohair Sebai

Table - 30
Percent distribution of children 0--5 years by level of haemoglobin in gms.

Com.	No. of Children	Haemoglobin gm %						Cumulative Readings		Total
		4+	6+	8+	10+	12+	14+	−10	10+	
A	95		3	15	41	36	5	18	82	100
B	123	1	12	22	43	21	1	35	65	100
C	90		10	24	50	12	3	34	66	100

* Reading in 10ths but chartered to nearest whole figure.

The distribution of the mean values of haemoglobin according to the age groups is shown in Table 31. In all three communities a relatively high value is observed in 0--1 age group, which decreases during the second year of life and rises slightly afterwards. This might be due to the depletion of the natural iron resources of infancy during the second year of life, due to the infant feeding practice.

X^2 test has been applied to differences in the Hg value of < 10 gm% between communities A and C. The difference is significant (p = <005)

Malaria: Malaria thin and thick smears from 135 school children were negative on microscopic examination.

In discussion with the key informants in Turaba, many of them mentioned "Homma Al Thuluth" –– the fever which comes every third day with chilling and ends with enlarged spleen. The fever was prevalent in Turaba twelve years ago at the time of "Al Haya" –– the rain. It was the great killer of children at that time.

Serological Tests

Treponema palladium FTA Test: Table 32 shows the results of FTA test for syphilis. Respondents of different age groups (except 0––4 years in Souq) showed reactions ranging from 6% to 25%.

At the end of the period of the study, I.V. blood was drawn from 3 males and 6 females from nomadic and semi-settled communities who came to the Health Center complaining of Shijar. FTA test was positive in all three males and in four out of six females. This could be taken as an indication that Shijar, which is widely known and commonly noticed by the natives, is a syphilitic disease.

Table - 31
Average values of Hg. in gms. among children by age group

Com.	No. of Children	Age in Years			All Ages
		−1	1–2	3–5	
A	95	10.9	10.5	11.3	11.4
B	123	10.9	9.3	10.4	10.2
C	90	10.5	9.1	10.2	10.1

Table - 32
Prevalence of seropositive reaction of FTA test for treponema by age group (Communities B & C combined)*

Com.	Age in Years	Resp.	Positive	
			No.	%
	0––4	13	––	––
A	5––19	16	1	6
	20+	20	5	25
	0––4	19	4	22
B, C	5––19	8	2	25
	20+	31	6	20

---

*   No Essential difference between the two communities.

None of the 4 children had specific complaint or clinical findings. Two of their mothers complained of rheumatic pains, and the third of chest pain. None of the other members of the three families had serological examinations.

Considering the high prevalence of the seropositive reaction among this young age group (22 per cent), the absence of clinical signs of congenital syphilis, the absence of suggestive history of syphilis among their mothers and being all Bedouin children, suggest that the disease is acquired by the children (endemic syphilis) rather than congenital.

Grin[30,] in his study of syphilis in Bosnia, Yugoslavia, attributed the disease as an endemic, non-venereal syphilis, caused by direct and indirect contact. He concluded that using of common domestic and household utensils often results in the appearance of infectious lesions in the oral region as the first symptoms. Franklin[25] also mentioned common utensils as a possible factor in the transmission of the treponema which penetrates the mucous membrane. In a study of syphilis conducted by a W.H.O. team in Asir province, West Saudi Arabia, they indicated that the syphilitic infection is prevalent in the area because of the socioeconomic and sanitary status of population, social habit, and the use of common eating and drinking utensils. They concluded that the disease is an endemic treponematoses[27].

Guthe[31] mentioned Saudi Arabia as one of the "islands" of endemic syphilis, in the Mediterranean region. He also attributed the transmission of the disease to common utensils such as drinking vessels. Hudson[37] described endemic syphilis (Bejel) as a "contagious, non-venereal, innocent syphilis of Bedouin children".

From the previous and other studies which describe endemic syphilis in its various names, such as 'Bejel', 'Sijar', 'Mabrook' and Ifringi', as a disease of Bedouins, we might conclude that the disease in Turaba is endemic syphilis. With all conservative precautions regarding the small number of serological tests and the shortage of evidence, some observation might support this latter conclusion.

1. Shijar is a disease of Bedouins.

2. Moral code among Turaba people is very strict against any extramarital sexual contact. However, a few cases of gonorrhoea among young unmarried men were observed in Souq (community A).

3. The four cases found in B and C with seropositive reactions are nomad children living in tents. Indications suggest that it is acquired rather than congenital syphilis.

VDRL Test: Due to the lack of a sufficient amount of sera, VDRL test was run on 82 samples of the sera. The agreement between the two tests (FTA and VDRL) is as follows:

Co-positivity	=	39%
Co-negativity	=	100%
Overall agreement	=	85%

Buck[9], in his study in Ethiopia, by comparing the two tests found a higher co-positivity (69%), a lower co-negativity (77%), with a less overall agreement (74.6%). The prevalence of malaria and leprosy among his population makes the comparison between the two studies difficult.

Fungal Diseases: The sera were examined for fungal antibodies.

Complement Fixation Test

Blastomycosis. Six out of 50 sera samples (12%) from community A were found positive for blastomycosis antibodies (titer 1:8––1:32).

Text books refer to blastomycosis as confined largely to North and South America[11]. A few cases were reported in Africa and other parts of the world[49]. In a discussion with Dr. John Binet, Mycologist, National Institute of Health, Bethesda, he suspected that the reported serological results were due to a cross reaction mechanism with other agents such as streptococci, histoplasmosis or coccidioidomycosis. Kaufman, from the Communicable Disease Center in Atlanta, mentioned that the serological procedures for diagnosis of North American blastomycosis are the least reliable of the fungal serologic procedures currently in use[43]. He mentioned also the possibility of the serological cross reaction with other agents, as tuberculosis, sarcoidosis and malignant disease.

Histoplasmosis (mycelian antigen). A serum sample of a two year old girl from Souq showed positive results of histoplasmosis antibodies (titer 1:8) as well as blastomycosis antibodies (titer 1:32). According to Kaufman[43], compliment fixation test of 1:8 is presumptive evidence of histoplasmosis, yet a lack of immunological response does not exclude histoplasmosis.

Histoplasmosis (yeast antigen) and coccidioidomycosis test were both negative.

Agar Gel Precipitation Tests: All were negative for the previous antigens.

In the light of the previous discussion and the unreliability of the blastomycosis serological test, we might conclude that histoplasmosis and antigens related to blastomycosis exist in Souq. This does not exclude the possibility that communities B and C might have histoplasmosis and a blastomycosis related agent, or for all communities to have blastomycosis.

Cholera Vibriocedal Antibodies: 98 samples of sera were examined for cholera vibriocedal antibodies. Of 41 samples of sera examined from Souq, 27 (65%) showed positive results for Ogawa strain, Enaba strain or both. Among 57 samples of sera examined from communities B and C, 32 (56%) were positive. In Souq 15 sera (55% of total positive sera) had a titer of more than 620, while in communities B and C 12 sera (36% of total positive sera) showed the same titer.

Historically no cholera has been reported in Mecca (the possible port of entry of cholera to Hejaz area in West Saudi Arabia) since 1912[68.] This would tend to exclude the existence of clinical or even subclinical cases which might be found in endemic areas.

The possibility for the prevalence of cholera antibodies among the examined population are:

1) previous vaccination

2) infection with nonspecific antigen.

Intestinal Parasites: Table 33 shows the results of the stool examination of children from Souq and communities B and C combined.

Table - 33
Percent distribution of children 0—5 years with intestinal parasites (Communities B & C combined)

Comm.	Number	With Infection	E. coli	N. nana	G. lamblia
A	87	40	19	15	14
B, C	99	43	20	16	26

Two pathogenic organisms, H. nana and G. lamblia, beside E. coli, were found. Approximately half of the children in both communities were infected by one or more of the organisms. Seven children in Souq and 17 children in B and C had multiple infections. All children less than 1 year old were negative.

No apparent aggregation of cases in individual households was observed. Children in 42 houses in all communities (with 2 or more children per house) were examined for intestinal parasites. In 11 of these households (26%) more than one child was positive, in 20 households (48%) one child was positive and the other was negative, and in 11 households (26%) both children were negative.

E. coli is almost equally prevalent in both communities. Although it is a none pathogenic organism, its presence is concrete evidence that the host has ingested faecal material.

Two school children living in Alawa complained of blood in the stool, and on stool examination Schistosoma mansoni eggs were revealed. Alawa village, 5 miles from Souq, is a known endemic focus for Schistosoma mansoni. In the summer of 1965, in a screening survey for schistosomiasis in Turaba, 32 stools were collected from Alawa children. Fourteen were positive on direct smear and an additional 4 on sedimentation of the entire stool[1].

The results of the stool examination in our study were felt to be on the low side. The collected samples were preserved in MIF stain (Merthiolate-Iodine Formalin) for three months before they were examined. This could have affected the results.

Rectal Swabs: Forty-four rectal swabs were examined bacteriologically. None of the material was positive for Shigella and Salmonella organisms. The absence of Shigella and Salmonella does not seem to be contradictory to the prevalence of diarrhea among the children under the study. Many cases of the acute diarrhea usually lack a definable infectious agent.

Tuberculin Tine Test. Fig. 6 shows the results of the Tine test, by age group and sex in 269 persons in community A and 118 persons in communities' B and C combined. Communities B and C show a higher prevalence of positive reactions (2mm and more) than community A among age group under 19 years, and more or less a similar prevalence among age group over 20 years. Females in both communities have a higher prevalence than males in age group under 19 years and less prevalence among age group over 20 years.

Maclennan[50] in his study among nomadic tribes in Jordan in 1935, using intradermal tuberculin test (Monteux), found the prevalence of Tuberculin positive reactions among children 5––15 years of age varied from 12.8% to 40% in different tribes.

Comparison between different communities is difficult not only because of the differences between communities, but also because of the greater sensitivity of the Mantoux test in which the reaction may be caused by infections with other types of unclassified myco-bacteria.

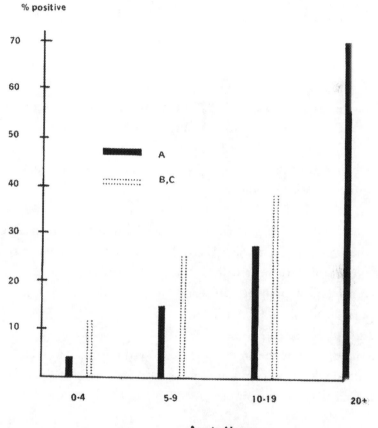

Figure 6. Percent of reactors to Tine test (2mm +) by age group (Communities B and C combined).

HEALTH KNOWLEDGE
AND ATTITUDES

Turaba is a changing community. Factors behind the change are:

1) Change in the Country –– The tremendous, rapid development and growth of the oil industry.

2) Local change –– The trend of Bedouin settlement increased with the drought. Even when the drought is over, We predict that the process of settlement will continue. The new geographic and social communication of Bedouins and villagers with the cities has created a new outlook on life for them.

Without understanding the present knowledge, attitudes and practice, it would be difficult to select and communicate new values to help the people adjust better to their changed environment.

Cultural barriers often make the introduction of new health concepts and practice difficult. We need to study the peoples' belief about the causes of disease and their priority values if we hope to introduce a new set of concepts. For example, nomads considered water to be safe and pure and not connected with disease. They regard a mosque as a far higher priority than a safe water supply. We must understand the social and cultural system in which the adult men eat together from the main dish leaving the leftovers for the women and the children, before we start to educate them on proper nourishment for their pre-school children. The people in Turaba use the doctor to treat their children for diarrhea and fever, while they might carry a child with dyspnea, who they believe is affected by Jinn, to the magic-religious man for treatment.

As Benjamin Paul wrote, "A thorough understanding of total ways and values and the importance of fitting new ideas into the existing cultural framework of the people were shown to be essential if lasting results were to be achieved"[7]. Hanlon[33] gave different examples from Bali and rural Burma to show how sudden and unplanned changes could be hazardous. "Popular health culture is the wine that fills the vessels. Ignoring this often results in spilling the new wine (scientific medicine) on the floor"[67].

Because of the length of the questionnaire, we limited the KAP (knowledge, attitudes, practice) study, as well as other areas of the study, to a sample of the households.

Eighty-four heads of the households were questioned about their knowledge of the etiology, treatment and methods of prevention of certain diseases: tuberculosis, mental sickness, shijar (syphilis), fever, diarrhea and body aches. Data about the subject were also collected through informal interviews.

In most of the KAP study, there is a little difference between the three communities. Whenever no difference appears, the results are discussed for the three communities combined.

Etiology of Diseases: The people believe in two main causes of diseases:

1) Supernatural power: God, Jinn and Evil Eye.

2) Physical agents: cold, heat and fatigue.

God is the primary cause of all disease. Still, for most diseases, there are intermediate causes such as Jinn or cold. Multiple causations are the pattern.

There is no concept of germs. Dirty water is not drunk because it is a nuisance rather than because it is hazardous.

Mental illness: Table 34 shows the belief in the causes of mental illness.

Table - 34
Distribution of beliefs in causes of mental sickness.

Com.	Resp.	God	Jinn	Fright	Walking/ Night	Evil Eye	Other
A	32	17	8	30	10	–	4
B	26	12	10	23	18	1	3
C	26	12	6	24	16	2	6
Total	84	41	24	77	44	3	13

People in all communities believe in certain basics:

1. Diseases, as every other single event in the life –– catastrophe or good fortune –– can happen to a person only by the order of God.

   "Say nothing will happen to you except what Allah has written." -- Quran.

2. God has created cause for every event including disease.

Concerning mental disease, the vast majority of people of Turaba believe that, by the order of God, Jinn can cause mental illness. He, the Jenny, enters the body of a human being if the latter is frightened or if walking alone at night. There is no variation in their beliefs. People, however, varied in their response to the question. Some mentioned the primary cause –– God, others mentioned the immediate cause –– Jinn, and a third group mentioned the circumstances in which the Jenni entered the body, i.e., walking by the night or fright.

Bedouins believe that every human being has a companion Jenny from the opposite sex. Sometimes the Jenni falls in love with his human partner and tries to enter his body. As a result, mental sickness occurs.

Case History: Ghuzail, an 18-year-old girl from Esala, was mentally sick. Her brother took her to a Saiid in Alula, some 300 miles from Turaba. The Saiid is a man who has the power to "extract" the Jinn from their victims. He either has studied the "Book of Jinn" or has a Jenny brother who tells him the secrets of Jinn. The Saiid tied the girl's big toes and thumbs with cloth, read her some verses from Quran and then beat her severely. A crying voice –– a man's voice –– came from inside the girl asking for forgiveness. The Jenny, after being beaten, admitted that he had been in love with the girl for a long time. One day she was milking her goat, and a dog suddenly howled behind her. She became frightened and agitated. At this moment the Jenny entered into her body. The Jenni was forced to leave the girl's body by the order of the Saiid, and Ghuzail got cured. "Tradition healers use primitive psychotherapy and spiritualism which definitely helps". (Murdock)[55].

It is interesting to note the similarities of different cultures. In Ecuador 48 school children were asked if they would consult a Curanduo for specified illnesses. Ninety-eight per cent of them would consult a Curanduo for freight (a magical, perhaps mental, disease) while only 4 per cent would consult him for tuberculosis (Foster)[24]. Evil eye was mentioned by three persons. However, it can cause other diseases such as epilepsy, apathy or severe sickness.

Tuberculosis: Table 35 shows the causes of tuberculosis as interpreted by the people in the three communities.

Table - 35
Distribution of perceived causes of tuberculosis.

Com.	Resp.	God	Contagious	Sun and/or Cold	Fatigue	Insufficient Food	Dirt	Don't Know	Other
A	32	7	20	10	1	9	–	2	7
B	26	6	14	16	4	8	3	3	3
C	26	19	11	10	2	6	4	2	5
Total	84	32	45	36	7	23	7	7	15

As in mental diseases, TB is believed to be caused by God, through direct causes. Nomadic people mentioned God as the cause of the disease more frequently than any of the other causes. On the other hand, more of the settled people mentioned contagion as the cause. Sun, cold, fatigue and insufficient food are thought to cause the disease either directly or through lowering the resistance of the body. Nobody mentioned germs.

As in mental disease, no apparent difference exists between the three communities.

Fever, body aches and diarrhea: Table 36 shows the causes of fever, body aches and diarrhea. There was essentially no difference in response within the three communities. The only exception was in body aches, where only one person from Souq against eight persons from the nomadic community mentioned Shijar as its cause. Regarding diarrhea, 9 persons, mainly from Souq, mentioned other causes as variations of food or indigestion, but no one mentioned a specific cause such as germs or contamination of water. Four said that fever is caused by malaria.

Table - 36
Distribution of perceived causes of fever, body aches & diarrhea (Communities combined).

	Respondents	Causes
Fever	81	Sun and/or Cold – 60, Fatigue –– 36, Exposure to endemic area –– 11, Other –– 8
Body Aches	82	Sun and/or Cold –– 66, Fatigue –– 64, Shijar –– 13, Other –– 12
Diarrhea	84	Overnight food –– 44 Overeating –– 10, Undercooked food –– 78, Other –– 9

Except in a few instances, the theory of cold and hot humors does not appear to play an important role in thinking. The Greek theory developed by Empedocles (490—430 B.C.) says that health is maintained by the harmony of the humors: the hot and the cold, the moist and the dry, is still popular among people in the cities.

Multiple causation and lack of specificity or scientific reasoning are the main features of the beliefs in the three communities. Their sources of information are sharp observation, long experience and personal communication, rather than regular education or mass media programmes.

Common and Fatal Diseases: One hundred and thirty three persons were asked what they thought was the most common disease in their community. The answers of the three communities combined are as follows:

Whooping Cough	72%
Measles	70%
Aching Pains	66%
Cough	48%
Shijar	33%
Diarrhea	14%
Fever	14%
Tuberculosis	10%
Other	18%

Essentially there is no difference between the three communities.

Although whooping cough, measles and cough are rated first, diarrhea (with actual high prevalence) is rated in the sixth place. Apparently, they consider it as a natural condition rather than a disease.

Table 37 shows the most fatal diseases among children as mentioned by the interviewees.

Table - 37

Percent distribution of people mentioned illness as fatal to children

Comm.	Resp.	Whooping cough	Measles	Cough	Fever	Diarrhea	Other
A	30	80	87	47	7	27	17
B	58	91	83	34	3	12	21
C	47	91	85	36	11	6	17

Again, respiratory diseases rated first, and diarrhea rated lower –– actually the lowest in the nomadic community.

Five diseases: whooping cough, measles, smallpox, tuberculosis and Shijar are considered infectious. All of these are thought to be transmitted by coming into contact with the patient either by sitting, eating or drinking with him. Whooping cough, in addition, could be transmitted to a child by hearing another child whooping. Shijar is transmitted from the mother to her infant baby through breast milk.

Smallpox, whooping cough and measles give permanent immunity "exactly like vaccine". "If you put a man who previously received smallpox among forty patients with the disease, he will not catch it".

Smallpox is the most dreaded disease. It not only kills, but equally disastrous, it might result in sterility in a man. The next most dreaded disease is whooping cough, which is the greatest killer of children.

One of the questions we asked was: "How could disease be prevented". The answer in many cases, "Nothing. Good will keeps us safe". Whenever a definite answer is given, it is usually to avoid the cause of disease.

We asked the people how tuberculosis could be avoided. Sixty two out of 84 in the three communities (73%) said by avoiding the patient. A close observation of their life, however, denotes that they behave differently. They eat, drink and come into close contact with a known patient of tuberculosis, "and God keeps us safe".

The heads of the households were asked about their health demands. "What do you want the government to do in order to improve the health conditions in your community?" In all our questions about demands we used the phrase "What do you want the government to do for you". The concept of community participation is not yet a part of their thinking. The percentage distribution of the answers is recorded in Table 38.

Table - 38
Percent distribution of respondent's health demands

Comm.	Resp.	None	Hospital	Health Center	Better Care in H.C.	Other Specific	Other Non-specific
A	59	5.1	89.8	1.7	5.1	1.7	5.3
B	106	7.5	11.3	68.3	7.5	1.9	6.6
C	88	6.8	14.8	73.9	5.9	1.1	8.0

Every group asked for its immediate needs. Almost 90% in Souq asked for a hospital. Almost 80% in the semi-settled and the nomadic communities asked for a health center (five in community C asked somewhat more realistically for mobile units). Six per cent in all communities asked for better care. People from Souq defined better care as an X-ray unit, surgical department and hospital beds. Those from the semi-settled and the nomadic communities asked mainly for more injections and better care from the doctor. Only four persons in all communities. asked about specific measures –– water purification, health education and vaccination.

In an open-ended discussion with the nomadic and the semi-settled people in communities B and C, we asked what they would most want the government to establish in their community. The constant answer was a school, a health center and a mosque. The priority setting was dependent on age. Young people rated school first and mosque last. Old people rated in the opposite direction. The health center was the second priority in almost all cases.

It seems to be a transient stage for the people in Turaba in their logical reasoning about their health demands. In early 1940, the people were reluctant to accept the health center services. At the present time, the health center is one of their priorities. They are not yet in the stage of asking for real public health programmes.

HEALTH PRACTICE

The health services available to the people of Turaba are of two types:

I   the Health Center

II folk medicine provided by native practitioners.

I The Health Center

The Health Center, a division of the Development Center, is composed of a professional staff consisting of a physician (Pakistani), pharmaceutical assistant (Pakistani), sanitarian assistant (Saudi), male nurse (Jordanian) and female nurse (Pakistani).

The services of the Health Center are mainly curative. The out patient load is between 90 to 110 patients a day (most of the patients are from Souq and Alawa). On average, the physician usually spends about two minutes with each patient. There are six beds at the Health Center which are used for emergency cases. No laboratory or X-ray services are available.

People from relatively remote areas cannot easily get to the Health Center due to the lack of regular transportation. Occasionally, adult males come to Souq for selling their products and shopping. It is not uncommon to see one of them asking the doctor in the Health Center for "medicines" for his son in

Elaba (45 km away) who has fever or abdominal ache. The Pakistani contract doctor must give the father medicine if he wants to live in peace in the area.

The physician keeps a log book in which registers the out patient cases. Diagnoses are recorded according to body system, which does not help in understanding the health problems of the area. There is incomplete birth registration and no death registration.

The male and female nurses are responsible for administering the injections (70% of the patients receive injections) and apply dressings when needed. In one four month period, the female nurse had conducted only seven deliveries in Souq and one in Alawa.

The sanitarian assistant, a position requiring a two-year training course in the health institution in Riyadh, is primarily responsible for preventative measures in Turaba. In the past two years, 880 cholera, 91 whooping cough and an unrecorded number of smallpox vaccination were administered. No other vaccinations were carried out.

The nearest general hospital is in Taif 140 km away. The physician refers an average of 10 cases per month to Taif, but in most instances patients go directly. It is a one way referral system in which the Health Center in Turaba does not follow-up the cases. In Taif general hospital, the tuberculosis hospital and mental hospitals there are no reliable records to tell the degree of utilization by the Turaba population.

In brief, the Health Center activities are confined to out patient services. There are no community based activities in health education, environmental sanitation, nutrition or maternal and child health programmes.

The educational and training background of the physician would appear to determine to a great extent his role as a diagnostician and a prescriber of drugs. The physician and his staff's main function seems to be to satisfy the demands of the people.

We asked the heads of households how much benefit they and their families were getting from the Health Center. The percentage distribution of the answers is shown in Table 39.

Table - 39
Percent distribution of perceived degree of benefits of the health center to the households.

Comm.	Resp.	Much	Moderate	Little or more	Total
A	60	15	60	25	100
B	101	4	34	62	100
C	87	6	25	69	100

We asked those who perceived little or no service what the reasons might be for this lack of services (Table 40).

Table - 40
Distribution of reasons for getting little or no service from the health center

Comm.	No. of households getting little or no service	Long Distance	The Cause Unsatisfactory Care	Never visited the H.C.
A	15	––	15	––
B	63	29	27	7
Could	60	21	25	14

Distance is a major determinant of use of the Health Center. From the Health Center records we find that out of 602 patients who visited the Health Center in one week, 518 (84%) came from areas within five miles of the Health Center. Many other studies have shown that the distance of the place of residence from the Health Center is a determinant factor in the utilization of health services[44, 51].

For the settled people, "unsatisfactory care" means mainly lack of X-ray unit or maternity beds and insufficient use of injections. For nomads and semi-settled it means primarily lack of injections. The doctor in Turaba refused to give unnecessary injections in the first two months of his assignment, but he finally gave in to popular demand.

II Folk Medicine and Native Practitioners

According to Elkins[31] "Aboriginal medicine men are far from being rogues, charlatans, or ignoramuses. They are men of high degree, men who have undergone tests and have taken degrees in the secrets of life much beyond that which ordinary men have a chance to learn. Their professional status and practice continue to be a source of faith and healing power to both themselves and their fellows".

There are various grades of native practitioners:

1. Highly specialized practitioners. These are six individuals; one magic religious practitioner who treats mental diseases, two bone setters who also perform minor operations and three general practitioners (internists) who treat various ailments using herbs and cautery. These practitioners are well known for their skills not only in Turaba but throughout the region. People as far away as Taif come to seek their advice and help.

2. There are about 18 persons well known locally for their knowledge and wisdom in diagnosis and treatment of diseases. Most of the time they are not paid for their treatment. They are considered the intermediate consultants in the lay reference system. Two of my key informants were among those practitioners.

3. Finally, there are many old and wise people in each community who are knowledgeable and are always willing to help and advice their neighbors and relatives.

A Bedouin mother might discuss the problem of her sick child with the grandmother and other members of the family. She might give the child Hawar (black pepper) if he has a cough, or Hawaij (seven different herbs collected from the native druggists and kept handy) if he has a fever. If the cough becomes severe or the fever persists, she would seek further help from the wise old people, then the semi-professionals and lastly the professionals.

The Health Center might come into the picture at any stage depending on the severity of the sickness, the age and sex of the patient and, primarily, the distance of the family from Souq.

We asked our respondents whether a doctor or a Bedouin practitioner is better in treating a group of diseases (Table 41).

Table - 41
Distribution of heads of households stating that selected diseases are treated better by the doctor

Comm.	No.	Cough	Diarrhea	Fever	Enlarged Lever	Enlarged Spleen	Gamba	Fracture
A	44	40	41	42	26	20	10	–
B	61	58	58	56	42	42	11	1
C	49	45	47	45	17	25	5	1
Total	154	143	146	143	85	87	26	2

We were surprised by the small difference in the attitude of people in the three communities. More than 90% in all communities favored a doctor for treatment of cough, diarrhea and fever. These are considered internal diseases, with physical not spiritual causes.

For enlarged liver and spleen, a lesser percentage (about 50%) in all communities favored a doctor. Although these are internal organs, they are palpable when enlarged. People often treat them by cautery and herbs. They can follow, with sharp observation, any change in their size, shape and tenderness.

In Gamba (a severe, sharp stretching pain in the side of the chest —— follows an acute, sometimes prolonged, disease of fever and wet cough —— presumably it is pleurisy) only about 16% preferred doctors.

Bone setting is the Bedouin practitioners' main specialty (only two people preferred the doctor to set a fracture). Even nowadays, in cities, when a bone fracture is mentioned, many people think immediately of calling in Al Badawi. They have a good reputation in their skill in setting bone fractures by splints. Dickson[17] in 1930 wrote, "Simple fractures are dealt with fairly satisfactorily with the Bedouins". People believe that gibs (plaster) rot the affected limb. The lack of orthopaedic specialists and, more importantly, proper post-operative medical care, are responsible for this well-founded belief.

Cautery is applied to young children for a variety of conditions, ranging from simple cough or prolonged crying to a severe case of convulsions.

I cannot draw a quantitative comparison between the three communities because cautery scarring drew my interest during the study. However, in all communities, at least every second child carries a cautery scar on his body.

The most extensive cautery scars are found on the negro children of Souq. Almost every child is cauterized, the average number being twelve. One child had 32 scars from cautery. The most common sites of cautery are the back, head, back and sides of neck and the extensor surfaces of the forearms and legs. Most cautery is done using the blunt end of a nail or a small branch of a tree. The tool is put into the fire until the end becomes red and it is then applied to the site of the complaint or a related organ (related by either blood or nerves).

Second to the negro children in the frequency of cautery are the nomad children and the least were the non-colored children of Souq.

The subject is very interesting. It deserves extensive study, not only for the epidemiology of the harmful effect of the act which certainly exists, but also for the physiological, pathological and the possible therapeutic effect. The long history (pre-Islamic) and the widespread use of cautery in urban and rural areas justifies the study.

Concerning the treatment of tuberculosis, 90% in all communities mentioned doctor and/or hospital as the preferred source of treatment. The disease is internal and obscure. People know little about its cause and pathology. It is dangerous, and more than that, in their long experience, its management by cautery and herbs apparently has not been successful. Hence a doctor or a hospital is preferable.

Native treatment of Shijar is another example of the conflict between the new and the old. Traditionally, Shijar is treated by drinking hot soup of wolf meat. Added to it are black pepper and plenty of animal fat and the patient is covered heavily. "The resulting sweat will expel the disease from the body". This is not unlike the fever treatment for syphilitic paresis in vogue a number of years ago in modern medicine. Recently, the trend is toward modern medical treatment. Thirty out of 32 (93%) in Souq said Shijar is better treated by a doctor; compared to 37 out of 52 (70%) in nomadic and semi-settled communities.

People recognize that measles comes in epidemics every two to three years (alternating with whooping cough) and they recognize that it gives solid immunity. It might kill children, but not as much as whooping cough. The child in the first seven days of the infection must taste from every available kind of food and he must ride a camel and an ass. If he is a breast-fed baby, his mother might do the above for him. For the next 40 days he must not eat any food that was not tasted in the first seven days or ride a camel or an ass if he did not do it in that period. Otherwise, he will get severely sick and might even die. After 40 days, he is allowed to eat and practice riding normally.

The health practice of the people in Turaba is largely shaped by the high degree of fatalism they adopt in life "Verily the physician, with his physics and his drugs, cannot avert a summons that has come. What ails the physician that he dies of the disease which he used to cure in time gone by? They died alike, he who administered the drug and he who took the drug, and he who imported and sold the drug and he who bought it". –– Old Arab Poetry.

One morning the Pakistani female nurse came to me with a native man whose wife had delivered that morning and had retained the placenta. In such a case no one is willing to interfere. The doctor (who happened to be on two days leave in Taif) would not have interfered. To avoid administrative and cultural problems, he never examined a lady vaginally. The female nurse would not dare interfere in what she felt was a complicated case. Traditionally, the people do not interfere with the process of delivery. No attempt is ever made (according to all whom I interviewed) to put a hand in the vagina of a delivering mother or even pull the child out. That morning it took me a fairly long time to convince the family to take the patient to Taif. They had refused saying, "God will save her, or she will die". Finally they agreed. We arranged a place for her and a companion in the daily car leaving Turaba before noon. At 5:00 p.m. I was told that the lady was still in Turaba, for the relatives changed their minds about taking her to Taif. The woman was in a state of shock. We gave her general anti-shock therapy and the female nurse, under what I had assumed was my responsibility, delivered the placenta.

Jassar from Esala is a 40 year old tuberculosis patient. He was admitted to Taif TB hospital for six months of treatment. Last year he was discharged as improved. They gave him PAS and "Ramfon" (Rimifon) and asked him to come back after one month for a general check-up. He never returned. He lost the slip of paper he was given and, moreover, he was busy. He is still coughing, but he takes a tablet whenever he has a headache, fever or feels weak. The proper attitude toward long-term treatment and the ability to learn are hindered by the lack of health education and proper follow-up.

The attitude toward vaccination is no longer negative as described by Dickson[18] in the thirties. It has become acceptable and even demanded in Souq, and to a lesser extent in semi-settled areas where some cholera and smallpox vaccination has been performed. In nomadic areas, the people are still not definite about wanting vaccination. "If the others will take it, I will".

CHAPTER III

TURABA
THE PRESENT 1981

A PROFILE OF
CHANGING TURABA

A visit was paid to Turaba in June 1981 to observe changes in health and health services and to assess the health services system and where it stands in contributing to the promotion of the health of the people.

No reliable demographic data is available for Turaba as expected in a community with a continuous mobility, settlement and migration back and forth to cities. The estimated population of Turaba is 45,000 people (compared with 30,000 in 1967), 20% of whom are still nomadic Bedouins.

Almost every aspect of life has changed in Turaba since the author's last visit. Souq, the main village, is unrecognizable for it has become a small modern town. The mud houses have been replaced by concrete buildings and have increased tenfold in number. The dirt roads have become asphalt streets and the half dozen small shops have been replaced by several modern markets. Electricity, telephones and color television sets are now a feature of almost every house.

Changes abound in the small settlement areas (Hejar) around Souq. They have increased in number and size, most are now accessible by asphalt roads and most of the mud houses and huts have been demolished and replaced by modern concrete buildings.

The most amazing changes have taken place in the desert. A Bedouin family, although still living in a tent, uses Butane gas for cooking and may own a small pick-up truck, usually driven by the housewife or her daughter. The Bedouin woman is probably the only woman driver in Saudi Arabia. A Bedouin herdsman feeds his herd with inexpensive barley which is subsidized by the Government. He also brings water in tanks to his location, and his livestock is taken to the market in a Mercedes truck. As a result he does not need to roam around as much as before looking for water and grass.

In general the average income of the family in Turaba has increased several folds over the last fifteen years. The family may have more than one source of income including farming, trade, government employment, animal husbandry (goats, sheep and camels), social security and financial support from young adults working in the cities.

The sudden economic improvement in Turaba, as in most parts of the country, started in the mid 1970's triggered by the tremendous increase in oil prices. In 1976 the Government also initiated a system of giving free loans of up to SR 300,000 to landowners in Turaba for the building of houses. In five years over 2,500 concrete houses were built, and 1,500 more are planned within the next two years. Other factors contributing to the process of economic development were: the establishment of a 140 km asphalt road to Taif, the introduction of electricity and telephones to Souq, and in the last two years an increase in the rate of rainfall after a long period of drought.

The economic improvement has been accompanied by social changes. In the late 1960's there were four schools for boys and one for girls. Now there are 17 boys' schools, and three girls' schools, and more are planned. Adult education for both men and women is in the process of development.

The social change shows itself in Ergain, a small settlement area (Hejrat) established in the late 1960's. The 100 or so mud houses and huts have given way to over 300 block and concrete buildings.

The people of Ergain, with the guidance of their wise old Sheikh Menahi Al Gharmool, have built two small one storey buildings –– one a school with a teacher provided by the Department of Education, and the other a dispensary, for which they are requesting a physician from the Department of Health. A co-operative committee was established and currently runs a bakery, grocery, petrol pump and a small generator which supplies electricity six hours a day to 30% of the houses. The people themselves helped in paving parts of the 20 km rough and rocky road to Souq.

Eating habits have changed. Rice and bread still constitute their staple food, but an average family can now purchase meat (which for them is the most precious food "it maintains health and gives power and vitality") or chicken almost every day. Milk, butter and dates are produced locally in sufficient quantities. Eggs and vegetables are available but seldom consumed as their nutritional values are not recognized. In the local grocery more than one brand of powdered milk is available for baby feeding, for the villagers a sign of modernization. A phenomenon observed in other developing societies[10,81].

People are becoming more orientated towards "modern medicine" but health services are still not easily accessible (more than 80% of the attendants of Souq Health Center come from a radius of 10 km). The people of Ergain, as in the case in the rest of Turaba, still seek folk medicine for many of their ailments, especially for Bedouin practitioner diseases such as bone fractures and mental diseases.

Fifteen years ago their main demands from the Government were simple, a dispensary staffed by a nurse, a boys' school and a mosque. Their demands at present are an asphalt road to Souq, a bridge over the wadi (the water bed separating Ergain from the main road to Turaba) a doctor to staff the health center, public electricity and a girls' school. According to their Sheikh, "out of ignorance and prejudice we resisted for years the opening of a girls' school in our Hejra, but now we ask for it because we see its relevance in the life of our women".

This socio-economic development has most likely led to an improvement in the health of the people in general and the young children in particular through improved nutrition, housing and education. It has its adverse aspects, such as the increase in the number of road accidents, artificial feeding for babies and the increased pressure of life.

The main question that remains to be answered is 'How has the Health Center contributed to the improvement of the health of the people of Turaba in the last fifteen years?'.

THE HEALTH CENTER

The health center in Turaba is still part of the Development Center (DC) which is composed of four units: Education, Social Welfare, Health and Agriculture. Each unit is sponsored and supervised by the corresponding ministry, and the Center as a whole is administered by the Ministry of Social Welfare.

In 1967 the Health Center in Souq was staffed by one Pakistani physician and four health assistants, a pharmacy assistant, a female nurse/midwife, a male nurse and a health inspector (the only Saudi member). The Health Center was the only provider of primary health services for the 30,000 inhabitants, whereas the secondary point of contact was at

Table - 42
The Staff of the Health Center in Souq, Turaba

No	Category of Personnel	Nationality[1]
3	Physicians (general practitioners)	Two Pakistanis (husband & wife) and one Egyptian
1	Dentist	Syrian
1	Midwife	Egyptian
2	Female nurses	Egyptians
3	Male Nurse	Palestinian
2	Pharmacy assistants	One Saudi and one Syrian
1	Laboratory assistant	Pakistani
1	X-ray assistant	Saudi
1	Health inspector	Saudi
1	Dresser	Yemeni

Taif, 140 km away by paved, but not asphalted road. The center was attended by an average of 95 outpatients per day, mostly coming from within a radius of 5 km; the services offered were exclusively curative.

In 1981 the Health Center in Souq is staffed by 14 health personnel (Table 42). The Center is the main provider of primary health care for 45,000 people and is attended by an average of 325 out-patients a day.

In addition to the Health Center in Souq there is a Health Center in Kara (6 km from Souq) and in Shir (25 km from Souq). Each is staffed by a physician

---

[1]   The 3 Saudis are graduates from the three Health Institutes in Saudi Arabia.

and three health assistants, one of whom is a Saudi and each Health Center is attended by 25 patients a day in average. Two other health centers are under construction in Souq; one is being built by the Ministry of Health (with 30 beds), and the other is private. Both are due to be open within the next six months. The nearest hospital is still in Taif, now connected to Turaba by 140 km asphalt road. Each one of the three functioning health centers in Turaba reports directly to the regional Director of Health Services in Taif.

In summary, the 45,000 inhabitants of Turaba are medically served by three health centers staffed in total by five physicians, one dentist and 16 health assistants. This gives a ratio of one physician to 9,000 people (compared to 1 to 1,450 in the Kingdom of Saudi Arabia); one dentist to 45,000 (1 to 26,000 in the Kingdom) and three health assistants to one physician (2.5 to 1 in the Kingdom). Of all the 22 personnel there are only 4 Saudi Health Assistants.

The functions of the Health Center in Souq will be described under two headings: curative and preventive aspects.

A. Curative Aspects

1787 patients attended the Health Center during the week preceding the study, a daily average of 325 (an average of 108 patients per physician per day). In addition, 17 patients are seen daily by the dentist. 15% of the patients are expatriate (Egyptians, Pakistanis, Indians and Yemenis), mostly unskilled laborers.

Table 43 shows the distribution by age group and sex of the 1,787 outpatients attending the Health Center during our sample week. The proportion of males to females is almost equal. The under 5 year old age group constitutes 16.8% of the total, which is rather a low figure in a community where the under 5 age group makes up approximately 20% of the population and is considered a risk group.

A patient coming to the Health Center may select his/her doctor as there is no registration, record system or screening. 80% of the females go to the lady doctor, whereas all male patients (over 5 years) go to the male doctors.

The two male physicians were observed for three hours in their clinic. The average time spent by each one of them seeing a patient was one minute and one second. The doctor would listen to the complaint, put his hand on the wrist of the patient and occasionally touch his chest with the stethoscope. At the same time he enters the patient's name, age and diagnosis in his log book, writes the prescription and hands it over to the patient. The writing takes a good part of his time.

No patient was adequately examined since there was no couch, sphygmomanometer or thermometer in the examination room.

Table - 43
Distribution of 1,787 out-patients who attended the Health Center over one week by age and sex.

| | Age Group in Years | | | |
	— 5 years	5—15 years	15 years +	Total
Male	148	97	677	922
Female	152	96	617	865
Total	300	193	1,294	1,787

The diagnosis, or rather the impression of the physician, follows a symptomatic pattern. Table 44 shows the distribution of diagnosis of the 1,787 cases seen by the three physicians over a one week period. The differences observed between men and women in cardiovascular, eye and skin diseases are more likely to be differences in judgment.

Table 45 shows the drugs prescribed for these 1,787 patients over a one-week period. The average number of drugs prescribed for a patient is 3. Multivitamins, analgesics and antibiotics are freely dispensed; together they constitute 74% of all drugs dispensed (indiscriminate poly-pharmacy). Non-specific drugs such as hormones (mainly testosterone for old men seeking sexual vitality) and cortisone derivatives have a higher ratio compared to more specific drugs such as antidiabetics and hypotensives. Antibiotics (including penbritin, tetracycline and streptomycin) are dispensed frequently in rather small doses. A patient may be given one injection of antibiotics and two days supply of 8 capsules.

Table - 44
Distribution of diagnosis of 1,787 cases recorded collectively by 3 physicians over one week.

Diagnosis	Men	Women	Children (--5 yrs)	Total	%
Gastrointestinal diseases	65	122	55	242	13.5
Chest diseases	110	83	78	271	15.2
Cardiovascular diseases	5	23	--	28	1.6
Nervous system diseases	14	31	--	45	2.5
Eye diseases	65	25	21	111	6.2
E.N.T. diseases	50	60	50	160	9.0
Bone & muscle diseases	158	196	2	356	19.9
Skin diseases	85	28	38	151	8.4
Genito-urinary diseases	39	48	--	87	4.9
Infectious diseases	6	6	10	22	1.2
Common cold	98	41	15	154	8.6
Others	79	50	31	160	9.0
Total	774	713	300	1787	100.0

Three prescription sheets selected at random from the pharmacy, clearly show the indiscriminate dispensing of drugs:

1. Diagnosis: Conjunctivitis
Streptomycin 1 amp.
Aspirin 6 tablets
Eye ointment 1 tube

2. Diagnosis: Headache
Aspirin 6 tablets
Multivitamin 6 tablets
Buscobpan 1 injection

3. Diagnosis: Chronic Bronchitis
Streptomycin 2 amp.
Aspirin 8 tablets
Multivitamin 8 tablets
Aminophellin 8 tablets
Penbritin 250 mg 8 caps.

Table - 45

Distribution of drugs prescribed for 1,787 out-patients in one week

Forms

Items	Tablets	Injections	Other forms[1]	Total	%
Analgesics	1,054	—	147	1,201	21.8
Vitamins	831	515	89	1,453	26.0
Antibiotics & sulpha	640	223	575	1,438	26.1
Cortisone derivatives	128	14		142	2.6
Hormones	43	17		60	1.1
Antimalaria	19	32		51	0.9
Antidiabetics	3			3	0.05
Hypotensives	3			3	0.05
Others	589	165	428	1,128	21.4
Total	3,310	966	1,239	5,515	100.0

Injections are highly favored by most of the patients — "it goes directly to the blood". Colored injections and calcium bromate (for the warm sensation it gives) are also in high demand. The physician prescribes medicine in injection form (even as one ampule of streptomycin) to satisfy the patient or as one of the physicians put it "a psychological treatment for the patient". A Bedouin attendant can even get a Vitamin B complex injection prescribed for his sister who does not feel well at home.

The clinical work is backed by laboratory and radiological services, which, although available are not utilized effectively.

Of the 325 patients attending the Health Center per day the laboratory technician performed an average of 8 simple routine examinations: 3 urine, 3 stool and 2 blood.

Out of 287 specimens of urine examined over a period of 4 months, 20 (7%) were positive for albumen, and 11 (4%) were positive for sugar. 162 specimens of stool examined over two months gave the following findings:

	No	%
E. coli cyst	12	7
G. lamblia cyst	13	8
H. nana	18	11
E. histolatica cyst	10	6

The X-Ray technician processes 12 cases per day.

The dentist treats an average of 17 patients per day. Table 46 shows the distribution of 94 patients seen over one week according to the complaint and type of treatment. 17 (16%) of the attendants were children below 15 years of age, male to female ratio was 3 to 1.

Table - 46
Distribution of 94 dental cases seen over one week.

Diagnosis	Filling	Extraction[1]	Scaling	Antibiotics alone	Total
Gingivitis			4		4
Acute abscess				6	6
Dental caries	22	49			71
Root canal diseases		13			13

[1]Extraction is always accompanied by antibiotics.

According to the dentist the population of Turaba has a high rate of dental morbidity. A man or a woman at the age of 25 has a third of his/her teeth either missing or with caries. This is most probably because of the high consumption of dates, and lack of oral hygiene.

One more activity is carried out. The Health Center also takes care of emergency cases such as simple wounds, first degree burns or scorpion stings. The Health Center refers approximately 15 cases every month to Taif Hospital, however no follow-up of the cases or feedback from the hospital is ensured.

An inspector would come from the Department of the Regional Health Services in Taif for a 1––2 day visit two or three times a year for general inspection and to solve emerging administrative problems.

B. Preventive Aspects

The estimated birth rate in Turaba is 45 per thousand, i.e. 2,025 live births per year for a population of 45,000. By law, a child should receive full immunization against poliomyelitis, DPT and tuberculosis before a birth certificate is issued. Because a birth certificate is not usually needed until school entry at the age of 6, a busy or a dilatory father can delay its issue for years provided he pays a penalty of SR 10.

For the expected 2,025 newly born children in 1980, 640 birth certificates were issued from the Health Center in Souq, the only place from which birth certificates are issued in Turaba. Only 258 children had received complete doses of poliomyelitis and triple vaccines during the same year. This is 40% of the 640 registered new born and only 12.7% of the 2,025 expected new born.

There is no recording of the age at which a child receives the first or subsequent immunization since there are no individual cards for the vaccines. BCG was given to 772 children during the first week of life. No other vaccines were being given, except in 1980 a mass vaccination against meningitis was carried out.

In the Health Center's refrigerator we found an ample quantity of BCG and diphtheria vaccines which had already expired, as well as measles vaccines which would expire within the month.

Last year 208 pregnant women (average 17 per month) visited the Health Center for general complaints. Each had been seen by the lady doctor, who examined her blood pressure and ordered a urine test for sugar and albumen. No follow-up program was carried out.

The midwife is called eventually to attend the delivery of a woman at her home (a delivering mother is usually assisted by an old experienced woman relative or neighbor). Last year the nurse/midwife attended 279 deliveries at homes out of the 2,025 expected deliveries (14%). There were no deliveries at the Health Center. Although a few mothers would be expected to go to the Hospital at Taif, there are no records available to verify this.

No other forms of MCH activities such as health education, nutrition, early detection of cases, neonatal or postnatal care take place.

The doctors in the Health Center by law are not permitted to make home visits, although some hidden private practice does occur.

School health for boys is the responsibility of the school health department under the Ministry of Education. One single physician works in Turaba and is responsible for 17 boys' school with over 2,000 pupils. The physician pays one or two visits a year to each school. In that one day visit he makes a general inspection and treats the sick.

Environmental sanitation is the responsibility of the municipality. Even the cleanliness of the Health Center building and its surroundings does not come under the jurisdiction of the doctors in the Health Center or their assistants. The two sanitarian assistants' main responsibilities are to record the out-patient statistics and fill in official forms for the Ministry of Health. They eventually vaccinate children when accompanied by their fathers. Last year they participated in a programme of installing 160 latrines in the villages.

Schistosomiasis is a recognized problem in Turaba but its epidemiology has not yet been studied. In a survey carried out last year among an unidentified number of school children in Souq, 32 students were found positive for

Schistosoma mansoni. A Schistosomiasis control team from Taif visits Turaba every 4—6 months for general survey and treatment. At the time of our visit, the team was completing a 12 day survey (planned and operated by the team from Taif) which covered 700 individuals. The survey recorded 15 positive cases, all natives, with Schistosoma mansoni and one Egyptian laborer with Schistosoma haematobium. Patients were treated by the Schistosoma team with no reference made to the Health Center. 97 wells previously reported positive for Biomphlaria species and treated with molluscicides (Moltox) were re-examined at this time. 28 were positive, an indication of ineffective control measures.

Discussion

It is quite apparent that the work being done by the Health Center is simply curative, or even palliative treatment, and there is no tangible program contributing to the prevention of diseases or the promotion of health. The main function seems to be to answer the simple demands of the people rather than meeting their actual health needs.

The physician spends on an average one minute for each patient. This is no way enables him to reach a proper diagnosis, treatment plan or educate the patient.

The indiscriminate prescription of drugs, especially antibiotics, can bring more harm to the patient than good and is also a waste of resources. The Ministry of Health alone spends on running costs of the health service an estimate of SR. 518 ($. 157) per capita per year. About 20% of which goes on drugs. Such valuable resources could be utilized more efficiently, if directed to preventive measures.

The diagnosis, being based on symptoms and recorded according to the "body system" does not provide any indication of the prevalence of diseases.

The laboratory and X-ray units could be more effectively utilized and the emergency room lacks essential facilities. In spite of the time and facilities available to the dentist, 66% of his patients leave the clinic with extracted teeth.

Out of nine working hours a day required from the physician, he or she spends 2 hours performing clinical work. The physician might spend another 2 hours in carrying out necessary administrative work and handling emergency cases, a total of 4 hours per day (less than 50% of the designated time).

We can only assume that each of the other members of the health team performs primary duties for about 4 hours of his time as well. This time could definitely be better utilized in providing more efficient ambulatory care. The rest of the time could be directed to community-based activities to prevent diseases and to promote the health of the people. Time and effort could also be utilized to initiate community participation and co-ordination with other agencies.

The question is, why the time of the staff is not efficiently utilized. In my opinion it is the issue of productivity relevant to expectation –– of the health authorities, the physician, the health worker and the people, in the community.

First the expectation of the majority of people, or their demand, from the Health Center, is very simple: a physician to provide treatment (preferably injections) for their ailments. The gap between this demand and the actual health needs, including maternal care, health education, vaccination, nutritional program and environmental sanitation is quite wide.

The illiterate villagers and Bedouins in particular, do not expect the physician to be meticulous in his clinical examination, but would prefer him to be quick and sharp. I once had a private clinic in Riyadh and some of my patients used to become irritated by what seemed to them lengthy history taking and examination. An old relative told me once that in India there are doctors who can diagnose diseases by touching the patient's wrist or observing his gait. He was highly impressed. One of the most successful private physicians in the city of Riyadh has the reputation of seeing over 300 patients per day. The patients in Turaba expect their physician to be sharp and quick and self-sufficient without much need for diagnostic aids.

They also expect him to give injections, the form of medicine which "goes directly to the blood". In Turaba 15 years ago, a newly appointed physician insisted on denying the request of his patients for injections but he gave up after a while when he discovered that patients started to disappear from his clinic to seek the private consultation of the health assistant who had a full bag of injections.

People expect to be seen by the physician as their first point of contact, and this is what they received. This is, of course, not the best use of expertise. If the time of a physician is to be utilized to the maximum for the health of the society, it should be rationally balanced between treating the sick and promoting the health of the people. The bulk of the out-patients should be screened by appropriately trained and well supervised health assistants, but even the physician himself does not see things this way. In discussing the point with him, he raised the classic question, "what if the health assistant makes a mistake?" He, of course, ignores the fact that he is highly liable to commit mistakes by running his clinic in the present manner.

People in rural societies, unless they are oriented and educated, do not expect the physician to run any preventive medical program. In a small village in Asir the physician has never organized a regular immunization program during the 10 years he has worked in the village. Nevertheless when he was due to be transferred to the city, the villagers pleaded with the authorities to keep him in the village.

The expectation of the authorities from the physician and his staff is to meet the demands of the people. Saudi Arabia is a democratic country, where people can have direct access to the press, the Ministry of Health, the Crown Prince, or even the King. If a man or a woman feels that his demands are not justifiably met, he can take his complaints to the highest authority and ask for justice. So, satisfying the people and avoiding unnecessary complaints is in itself an important aim.

The authorities expect the physician to send a monthly out-patients attendance report, categorizing the diseases according to the body system. When a newly appointed physician sent his first report based on International Classification of Diseases of WHO, he was blamed by the authorities for being different and not following the rules.

The authorities do not expect the doctor to pay home visits, fearing that he may obtain money from patients, thereby depriving him of real contact with life outside the Health Center.

The physician's expectations from society, the health authorities, his aides and not least from himself, play the greatest role. His self-image as a diagnostician and a drug prescriber has already been defined for him by his medical education. The courses he studied in hygiene, preventive medicine or community medicine provided him with the knowledge but did not enable him to formulate a solid basis, or the capability, to establish preventive and promotive programmes.

As one of the physicians put it when I discussed with him the possibility of converting the present Health Center into one dealing with primary health care providing comprehensive health services: "Good. This will let us know about the activities" Strange! He did not see himself as part of the system. It is rather the responsibility of the health assistants. When I raised the point of the expired vaccines he responded by saying "vaccines and vaccination are the responsibility of the sanitarian assistant" and then he added "also the sanitation is his responsibility".

In many instances the expectation of an expatriate physician working in a foreign country such as Saudi Arabia is to establish himself financially before he returns back home. Nothing wrong with that, but the problem comes when he considers his stay in the country as a transient stage, which does not require him to identify himself with the people or with their problems.

In conclusion, the Health Center in Turaba has a minimum contribution to the promotion of health among the people. The main question still remains: how the situation can be changed in order to produce better Health Services. This is what we will try to answer in the next chapter, "Turaba: the future, 1990".

CHAPTER IV

TURABA
THE FUTURE 1990

A PLAN OF ACTION

R esearch in the field of health cannot be an end but rather a mean for change. If the previous two chapters on Turaba in the past and at present can work as a stimulant for thinking in the future, this chapter suggests a guideline for health services development. It is a preliminary plan of action for a Primary Health Care (PHC) model to develop health services in Turaba community by 1990.

This guideline is not intended to replace a rational detailed plan, as this is left for further discussion and dynamic thinking. Health planners, health providers, health professionals, technical people and representatives from the community should participate in the planning and implementation of the final program.

The proposed PHC plan could be seen as a conceptual model applicable, after modification, to other communities in Saudi Arabia and possibly abroad. Continuous evaluation and feedback should be integral parts of it's implementation.

The Plan of Action for PHC in Turaba

1. Objectives

—— To provide a comprehensive health care program (curative, preventative and promotive), designed to; (a) reducing morbidity and mortality and (b) improving the health status of the people.

—— To provide training and research opportunities for health personnel.

2. Functions

—— The provision of comprehensive and integrated health services to individuals, families and the community, including: curative services, health education, environmental sanitation, maternal and child health, nutrition, immunization and mental health.

—— Services should be carried out with the full participation of the community in identifying the problems, planning and programming, implementation, follow up and evaluation. This would develop an appreciation for the health services, better communication and understanding of the local values, self-reliance and mobilization of local resources.

—— Training programmes at both undergraduate and post graduate levels of medical students, doctors, planners, administrators and other health workers would enhance future developments.

—— Collection of base-line data and carrying out applied research for better understanding of the health problems and their ecological background, and to search for proper solutions.

3. Basic Considerations:

People:

—— There is no up to date census or demographic data available. The population is estimated at 45,000, 20% are Bedouins; the annual population growth is about 3.6%. The settlement of Bedouins, migration to cities and importation of foreign laborers is a continuing process. Children below 15 years of age constitute 48% of the population.

—— IMR is estimated at 100 per 1000 live births ranging from 80/1000 in the main town to 120/1000 among Bedouins.

—— The basic health problems are related to inadequate sanitation, lack of health education and infectious diseases.

—— Turaba is developing socio-economically. This will lead to a change in lifestyle, better housing, nutrition and education.

Primary Health Care:

—— Primary Health Care is neither a second class solution for poor countries nor a cheap method to apply. It is rather the challenge of meeting the basic and essential needs and demands of the people in an integrated and comprehensive way.

—— All member states of the World Health Assembly who endorsed the Resolution on Health for All by the Year 2000, confirmed PHC as the central thrust.

—— It is applicable in developed as well as in developing countries, and affluent as well as poor societies.

4. Requirements for the Implementation of the Plan

High Authority support and commitment
Financial resources
Administrative reforms
Health personnel
Community participation
Intersectorial co-ordination
Link to a medical school

High Authority Support and Commitment

The coverage of the Kingdom by a network of Primary Health Care has already been considered as one of the main goals of health sector in the third Five-Year Plan (1400–-1405 A.H. = 1980–-1985 A.D.). What is needed is a common understanding of the objectives and functions of PHC among the high authorities.

In the country at the present time there are 380 Health Centers (staffed by physicians) whose functions are mostly curative. It is expected that by 1985 the number of Health Centers will be 505 (64% increase).

To turn all or the majority of these Health Centers into comprehensive health care centers is not possible. A more realistic plan is to start with selected PHC units as a model, to help in defining the best formula for Saudi Arabia, prior to the propagation of the idea to the rest of the country during the next one or two decades. The proposed PHC in Turaba could serve as one of these pioneering models. The other models could be established in other areas of the country, preferably attached to the medical schools.

The understanding, support and commitment of the health authorities, particularly in the Ministries of Health, Planning and Finance in Riyadh and at the regional level are essential for the success of the plan. This support would facilitate both the provision of adequate financial resources to the PHC as well as Administrative reform.

Financial resources

The budget allocated to the health services (except military health) is SR. 13.6 billion for the year 1401–-1402 A.H. At least 80% of the MOH budget presently goes to hospital services, whereas almost 80% of the health problems in a developing country like Saudi Arabia could be adequately be met at PHC level. What is required is a correction of the disproportionate allocation of the health budget. The additional resources for PHC should be utilized not only in increasing the number but even more important to improve their quality through:

a) Improving the quality of the health personnel and preparing them to meet the health needs of the people.

b) Designing and building a new type of health centers which suit the purpose. Most of the present health centers and dispensaries are accommodated in rented buildings.

The health team in a village in Qasim when moved to a newly established health center, made an improvement in its activities over the health team in an adjacent village which remained in the old mud house[75].

c) Conducting operational research into health administration, Administration is the bottle neck in the success of health projects.

The community itself should contribute to the PHC both through donations and also paying fees for services. The additional income should be utilized for continuing improvement of the center.

Administrative reform

The recent economic prosperity in the Kingdom has led to changes in almost all aspects of life: education, urbanization, housing and so forth. The health services have expanded about 2.5 times in the last decade. A new way of thinking should be adopted to handle the changes in health needs and demands.

In 1978 over 200 physicians attended two week courses in community medicine. Apparently the courses did not change their practice since they went back to work within the same system and the same environment. At the end of one of the courses, the 25 participants were asked: What does a PHC physician needs to improve his work? The majority indicated that he needs a sense of belonging.

PHC in Turaba should be given adequate autonomy in a sense that the leading physician and his team should be involved in the planning as well as the operation of activities. This will give them a feeling of responsibility and self respect, and it should be done in accordance with a dual referral system which ensures standardization, supervision and follow-up from the Regional Director of Health Services in Taif.

Health Personnel

A major obstacle PHC is facing in Saudi Arabia is the quality of the health personnel. The physical resources are almost sufficient if utilized efficiently, and so is the number of health personnel, if appropriately used. The quality of most of the health personnel including their training, education, motivation, ability to communicate and leadership capacity needs to be improved.

The majorities of the health personnel in Saudi Arabia are and will remain for many years to come, expatriate. Many of them do not speak Arabic and are not oriented to the health ecology and health problems of the Kingdom.

In the case of Turaba the three physicians and the dentist are all expatriate which hinders their leadership capacity even if they have the quality. This stems mostly from the culture which expects the expatriate to follow the rules rather than to innovate. Two of the physicians are non-Arabs, a fact which limits their ability in communication with other health workers and the community.

One would expect from physicians working in a PHC set-up to be adequately educated in the areas of:

— Ecology of health, which interrelates between health per se and the socio-economic and environmental factors

— Primary health care-concept, philosophy, objectives and techniques

— The role of the physician as a leader, educator, clinician and health promoter

— The role of the community as a primary participant in the health services system

Unfortunately the classical system of medical education prevailing at the present time in most parts of the world does not sufficiently prepare physicians to play their proper role in PHC. The same would apply to the other members of the health team.

The strategy to overcome the problem could be carried out in two phases:

Short term plan:

i) Conducting refresher courses and on the job training for all catagories of health workers in the objectives, functions and activities of PHC.

ii) Better selection in the recruitment of personnel to the system.

Long term plan:

i) Establishing a school of public health in Saudi Arabia to train leaders in the health services system.

ii) Supporting and promoting the new trend in medical education, being realistically adopted by the present medical schools. The new trend calls for community based, problem solving approach.

Community Participation

This is an issue of an utmost importance. The community should participate in all the activities of the PHC, defining the problems, planning, implementation, follow-up and evaluation. Also it should contribute to its physical and human resources. School teachers and pupils, religious leaders and many other individuals and groups can be involved.

Section VII of the declaration of Alma Ata states that PHC "requires and promotes maximum community and individual self reliance and participation in the planning, organization, operation and control of Primary Health Care making fullest use of local, natural and other variable resources"[93.] The concept has also been highlighted in the preceding conference held in Halifax, May 1978 on "Primary Health Care: A Global Perspective, the Role of Non-Governmental Organization".

Seven countries participated in a study on "Country Decision Making for the Achievement of the Objective of Primary Health Care" indicated that community participation is vital for the success of PHC[86].

Turaba itself can give an example of the readiness of the people to participate in public projects. Ergain people under the leadership of their Sheikh donated two small houses for the school and the dispensary, paved part of the road to Souq, and introduced electricity to the Hejrat. Our experience in the field supports this self reliance attitude among rural communities. In Tamnia village the school children and their teachers contributed to the cleanness of their village[52]. In Qasim village school children and their teachers were activated to carry out a program of Trachoma control, health education and vaccination in their community[80]. In ARAMCO Medical Department, Saudi Arabia, a reduction of diarrheal diseases in children was achieved by the introduction of "day care" programs with the participation of the mothers[3].

Community participation can also be expressed by paying nominal fees for outpatient services. The government of Saudi Arabia is determined to provide her people with appropriate health care facilities. The principle of applying nominal fees for certain aspects of health services had already been accepted by the authorities in response to the first national development plan. It is expected to give better recognition of the health services from the part of the people, emphasize the contribution of the community and help in cutting off some of the unnecessary load on the health facilities. The income from the fees should be under the disposal of the Health Center to initiate community based projects and carry out general improvements.

Community participation in physical, human and moral forms, will build up self reliance, self identification with the health projects and a feeling of belonging. The village committee or likewise, if strong and motivated can give the initiative for community participation.

Sectorial Co-ordination

Health promotion is beyond the capacity of the health sector alone. Various government sectors such as the departments of agriculture and municipality should co-operate with the health sector. The Development Center with its four sections: health, agriculture, education and social welfare can work as a base for such co-ordination.

Link to a Medical School

The PHC will function as a base for training programmes in family medicine practice, health administration, and a wide range of preventive programmes. On-the-job training, short courses, symposia and conferences can be held for health personnel from the region.

The linking of the pioneering PHC centers with Medical schools would facilitate to a great extent the education and training programmes. Research will also be promoted. The idea of connecting PHC to educational institutions has been implemented successfully in Rockford School of Medicine, University of Illinois College of Medicine[66], University of Washington School of Medicine[28], Bu Ali Sina University, Hamadan, Iran[89], University of Glasgow[35] Hacettepe University Turkey[23] and in Kenya[20,21].

APPENDIX

Sample Size

During the preparatory phase of the study (1966) we tried to determine a sample size which would be large enough to detect a real difference of 30/1000 in IMR between the two communities (settled and nomadic) at 5 per cent significant level. (Bothc $\propto$ and β .05)

With the base IMR at 150/1000, the corresponding normal deviates become

$$Z_{\alpha} = 1.64 = \frac{D - 0}{\sqrt{\dfrac{(2)(.15)(.85)}{n}}}$$

$$Z_{B} = 1.64 = \frac{D - .03}{\sqrt{\dfrac{(2)(.15)(.85)}{n}}}$$

where D is the minimum observed difference required for a declaration of significance, and n is the number of exposed infants in each community. Solving for D and n produces n = 3,048 infants

n is an unreasonably large sample size.

During the pilot study in the summer of 1966, the Ministry of Labour and Social Welfare planned to provide us with three male and three female interviewers to participate in the study for a period of two months. Considering other limiting factors beside the number of personnel and time, such as the multiplicity of communities, disparity of houses, difficulty of transportation between communities, we figured that we would be able to study three hundred households. Actually we studied 314 households in addition to the twenty per cent replicate.

Here we are trying to determine the ability of our sample size to detect a real difference in the infant mortality rate (IMR) and 1––4 year age specific death rate (CMR) based upon the following considerations:

1. We are interested in comparing IMR and CMR in the two communities, the settled and the nomadic.

2. We assume (based on the pilot study) that

IMR = 150/1000

CMR = 25/1000

3. We are assuming that the two rates are statistically independent.

4. Because of the small sample size available, we are willing to merge the observed IMR and CMR into a single analysis of significance. Letting

$\propto$ I = risk of type I error with respect to IMR,
$\propto$ c = risk of type I error with respect to CMR,
$\propto$ t = risk of type I error in combined analysis,

we require

$$t = .05$$

and

$$\propto I = \propto c.$$

Then we require the results of both the IMR and CMR comparisons to be tentatively significant in order for ultimate significance to be declared in the combined analysis. Hence

$$\propto t = \propto I \propto c,$$

from which it follows that

$$.05 = (.23)^2.$$

Based upon these considerations, the resulting values of B were calculated under several circumstances. For example, in the event of a real difference of 30/1000 in IMR between the two communities, we found

$$Z\alpha = -0.74 = \underline{D - 0}$$

$$\sqrt{\frac{(2)(.15)(.95)}{50}}$$

from which

$$D = .0525$$

Then

$$Z_B = \underline{0.525 - .03}$$

$$\sqrt{\frac{(2)(.15)(.95)}{50}}$$

from which

B = .63

The other results of these calculations are summarized below.

Infant Mortality Rate

Difference between 2 communities/1000 (M)	B
30	.63
50	.51
70	.35
100	.25

Child 1––4 years old specific death rate

difference/1000	B
50	69.5
100	67

Conclusion: The sample size is still not large enough to assure identification of a realistic difference in the IMR and the CMR. Therefore we must look at multiple measurements, both quantitative and qualitative, noting the direction of difference, i.e., if the observed differences are in the same direction for several variables, the significance of the findings is increased.

BIBLIOGRAPHY

1. Alio, I.S. Epidemiology of Schistosomiasis in Saudi Arabia. Unpublished Dr. P. H. dissertation, Aramco, Saudi Arabia (1969)

2. Aramco Economic Department. Reports and abstracts from reports. Dhahran, Aramco. (Unpublished)

3. ARAMCO Epidemiology Bulletin. Aramco Medical Department, Dhahran, Saudi Arabia. June –– July 1974.

4. Ascoli, W. et al. Nutrition and infection field study in Guatemalan villages, 1959 –– 1964. IV: deaths of infants and pre-school children. Arch. Environ. Health, 15: 439 –– 449, 1967

5. Baker, T.D. Problems in measuring the influence of economic levels on morbidity. Am. J. Public Health, 56: 499 –– 507, 1966.

6. Banoub, S. Primary Health Care in Qasim. A profile of two villages in the Qasim region. Sebai, Z.A. Ed. Saudi Medical Journal Monograph Ser. (In press).

7. Benjamin, P. Health, Culture and Community; case studies of public reactions to health programs. New York, Russell Sage, 1955.

8. Briggs, L.C. Tribes of the Sahara. Cambridge (MA), Harvard University Press, 1960. p. 174.

9. Buck, A.A. & Spruyt, D.J. Seroreactivity in the venereal disease research laboratory slide tests and the fluorescent treponemal antibody test. Am. J. Hyg., 80: 91 –– 102, 1964.

10. Carbello, M. Fertility regulation during Human Lactation. WHO Collaborative studies on breast-feeding. J. biosoc. Sci, Suppl. 4(1977), 83––89.

11. Davis, B.D. et al. Microbiology. New York, Harper Medical, 1973. p.p. 985 –– 986.

12. Dickson, H.R.P. The Arab of the desert; a glimpse into Bedouin life in Kuwait and Saudi Arabia. London, Allen and Unwin, 1959. p. 190.

13. Dickson, H.R.P. ibid. p. 144.

14. Dickson, H.R.P. ibid. p. 167.

15. Dickson, H.R.P. ibid. p. 172.

16. Dickson, H.R.P. ibid.

17. Dickson, H.R.P. ibid. p. 511

18. Dickson, H.R.P. ibid. pp. 505 –– 514

19. Dixon, W.J. & Massey, F.J. Introduction to statistical analysis. 2nd ed. New York, McGraw Hill.

20. Fendall, N.E. Paper presented at the Rural Health Conference of the South Pacific Commission, Tahiti, April 1963.

21. Fendall, N.E. et al. A national reference health center for Kenya. East Afr. Med. J., 40 (4), 1963

22. Filali, M. The project of Bedouin settlement in Saudi Arabia. (Unpublished) (In Arabic). Ministry of Labor and Social Welfare, 1964.

23. Fisik, N. Professor of Community Medicine, Hacettepe University, Ankara. Personal communication.

24. Foster, G.M. Use of anthropological methods and data in planning and operation. Public Health Rep., 68: 841 –– 857, 1953.

25. Franklin, H.T. Communicable and infectious diseases; diagnosis, prevention and treatment. St. Louis, C.V. Mosby, 1964. pp. 691 –– 702.

26. Gersovitz, M., Madden, J.P. and Smiciklas-Wright, H. Validity of the 24 hour dietary recall and seven day record for group comparisons Journal of the American Dietetic Association. vol 73. July 1978.

27. Ghoroury, A.A. The syphilis problem in Asir Province, Saudi Arabia. Bull. WHO 10: 691 –– 702, 1954.

28. Gordon, M.J. et al. Evaluation of clinical training in the community. J. Med. Educ., 52: 888 –– 895, 1977.

29. Gordon, ––. Weanling diarrhea. Am. J. Med. Sci., 245: 345 –– 377, 1963.

30. Grin, E.I. Endemic syphilis in Bosnia. Bull. WHO, 7: 1 –– 74, 1952.

31. Guthe, T. Die Bekampfung der Endimishen Syphilis in Entwicklungslandern. Arch. Klin. Exp. Dermatol. Ges., 219: 194 –– 210, 1964.

32. Haddad, N.A. Trachoma in Lebanon; observation on epidemiology in rural areas. Am. J. Trop. Med. Hyg., 14: 652 –– 655, 1965.

33. Hanlon, J.J. Principles of public health administration, 4th ed. St. Louis, C.V. Mosby, 1964.

34. Hanlon, J.J. ibid. p. 118. (Quotation from Elkins, A. Aboriginal man of high degree. 1944).

35. Hannay, D.R. & Maddox, E.J. The use and perception of a health center. Practitioner, 218: 260 — 266, 1977.

36. The Hashemite Kingdom of Jordan. Nutrition survey, April — June 1962. (Report by the Interdepartmental Committee on Nutrition for Jordan).

37. Hudson, E.H. Treponematosis in perspective. Bull. WHO, 32: 735 — 748, 1965.

38. James, W.P.T. Kwashiorkor and Marasmus: Old Concepts and New Developments. Proc. roy. Soc. Med. Volume 70 September 1977.

39. Jelliffe, D.B. Assessment of the nutritional status of the community. Geneva, WHO, 1966. (WHO Monograph Ser., no. 53).

40. Jelliffe, D.B. ibid. p.93.

41. Jelliffe, D.B. Infant nutrition in the subtropics and tropics. 2nd ed. Geneva, WHO, 1968. (WHO Monograph Ser., no. 29). pp. 27 — 37.

42. Joint FAO/WHO technical meeting on methods of planning and evaluation in applied nutrition programs; report. Geneva, WHO, 1966. (WHO Tech. Rep. Ser., no. 340).

43. Kaufman, L. Serology of systemic fungus diseases. Public Health Rep., 81: 177 — 185, 1966.

44. King, M.H. Medical care in developing countries; a symposium from Makerere. (1: 3) Oxford, Oxford University Press, 1966.

45. Lewin, K. Factors behind food habits and methods of change. Bull. Nat. Res. Counc., 108, 1943.

46. Lipsky, G.A. Saudi Arabia; its people, its solity, its culture. New Haven, H.R.A.F. Press, 1959. p. 48.

47. Lipsky. G.A. ibid.

48. Lipsky, G.A. ibid. p. 297.

49. Lythcott, G.I. & Edgcomb, J.H. The occurrence of South American blastomycosis in Accra, Ghana. Lancet, (1964) 1: 916 –– 917, 1964.

50. MacLennan, N.H. General Health conditions of certain Bedouin tribes in Trans-Jordan. Trans R. Soc. Trop. Med. Hyg., 29: 227 –– 248, 1935.

51. Mazen, A.K. The development of the rural health program of the U.A.R. United Nations conference on the application of services and technology for the benefit of less developed areas, October 1968.

52. Miller D.L. & Sebai, Z.A. Health Center in Khulais. In: Proceedings of the 5th Saudi Annual Medical Meeting, Riyadh University, Faculty of Medicine, 1980. (In press)

53. Molina, G. & Norm, I.F. Indicators of health, economy and culture in Puerto Rico and Latin America. Am. J. Public Health. 54: 1191 –– 1206, 1964.

54. Morley, D.C. et al. Heights and weights of West African village children from birth to the age of five. West Afr. Med. J., Feb. 1968.

55. Murdock, G.P. Anthropology and its contribution to public health Am. J. Public Health, 42: 7, 1952.

56. Murray, E.S. et al. Agents recovered from acute conjunctivitis cases in Saudi Arabia. Am. J. Ophthalmol., 43 (4, pt. 2): 32, 1957.

57. Muslim, 1: 48. (In Arabic)

58. Nelson, W.E. Textbook of paediatrics. 8th ed. Philadelphia, W.B. Saunders, 1964. pp 48 –– 49.

59. Neumann, C.G. et al. Nutritional and anthropometric profile of young rural Punjab children (In press).

60. Opitz, K. Die Medizin im Koran. Stuttgart, Verlag von Ferdinand Enke, 1906. p. 15.

61. Patai, R. Golden river to golden road; society, culture and change in the Middle East. Philadelphia, University of Pennsylvania Press, 1962. p. 84.

62. Patai, R. ibid.

63. Patai, R. ibid. p. 92.

64. Patai, R. ibid. p. 97.

65. Patai, ibid. p. 95.

66. Pittman, J. & Daniel, M.B. Undergraduate education in primary care; the Rockford experience. J. Med. Educ., 52: 982 –– 990, 1977.

67. Polgar, S. Health and human behavior; areas of interest common to the social and medical services. Curr. Anthropol., 3: 159 –– 205, 1962.

68. Pollitzer, R. Cholera. Geneva, WHO, 1959. (WHO Monograph Ser., no. 43) p. 63.

69. Proceedings of the XIV International Congress of Sociology, Rome, 1950, vol. IV. p. 1––18.

70. Puyet, J.H. et al. Nutritional and growth characteristics of Arab refugee children in Lebanon. Am. J. Clin. Nutr., 13: 147 –– 157, 1963.

71. Qur-an IV: 3

72. Qur-an II: 233.

73. Sebai, Z.A. Ed. Community health in Saudi Arabia: a profile of two villages in the Qasim region. Saudi Med. J. Monograph Ser. (In Press).

74. Saudi Arabia, Ministry of Finance and National Economy, General Statistics Office, 1977.

75. Sebai, Z.A. Ed. Community health in Saudi Arabia: a profile of two villages in the Qasim region. Saudi Med. J. (In press).

76. Sebai, Z.A. Health Manpower Development in Yemen Arab Republic. WHO assignment report, EM/HMD/359, 1976.

77. Sebai, Z.A. Health Manpower Development in Oman. WHO assignment report, EM/EMD/394, 1978.

78. Sebai, Z.A., Miller, D., Ba'ageel, H. Study of three Health Centers in Rural Saudi Arabia. Saudi Medical Journal, 1. No. 3, Jan. 1980.

79. Sebai, Z.A. Ed. Community health in Saudi Arabia: A profile of two villages in the Qasim region. Monograph Ser. Saudi Med. J. (In press).

80. Sebai, Z.A. Ed. ibid. (introduction).

81. Taha, S.A. Ecological Factors Underlying Protein-Calorie Malnutrition in an irrigated area of the Sudan. Ecology of food and nutrition 1979, vol 7, pp. 193--201.

82. Taha, S.A. The Prevalence and Severity of Protein-Calorie Malnutrition in Sudanese children. Tropical Paediatrics and Environmental Child Health. October 1978.

83. Taylor, C.E. et al. Eye infections in a Punjab village. Am. J. Trop. Med. Hyg., 7: 42 –– 50, 1958.

84. Third Development Plan, 1980 –– 1985. (Saudi Arabia) 1981.

85. Trowell, H.C. & Jelliffe, D.B. Diseases of children in the subtropics and tropics. London, E. Arnold, 1958. p. 194.

86. UNICEF/WHO. National decision making for primary health care. Geneva, WHO, 1981. (UNICEF/WHO JC 23).

87. United Nations. E/CN5/346/Rev. 1. Reference 5, diagram 1, p. 46.

88. United States, National Health Survey. Disability from specific causes in relation to economic status. Washington D.C., 1938. (Preliminary Rep. Sickness Med. Case Ser. Bull., no. 9).

89. Villareal, R. Health services and manpower development program, Iran, Hamadan and West Azerbaijan provinces. Geneva, WHO, 1977. (WHO Assignment Rep. EM/HMD/383).

90. Walpole, N.C. et al. Area handbook for Saudi Arabia. DA Pam. no. 550 –– 551: 50, 1966.

91. WHO expert committee on medical assessment of nutritional status. Geneva, WHO, 1963, (WHO Tech. Rep. Ser., no. 258).

92. WHO international standards for drinking water. Geneva, WHO, 1958.

93. WHO/UNICEF primary health care; report of the international conference on primary health care, Alma-Ata, USSR, 6––12 September, 1978.

ENGLISH BOOKS
PUBLISHED BY TIHAMA

* Tihama Economic Directory.

* Riyadh Citiguide.

* Banking and Investment in Saudi Arabia.

* A Guide to Hotels in Saudi Arabia.

* Surgery of Advanced Cancer of Head and Neck.
                    By F. M. Zahran
                    A.M.R. Jamjoom
                    M.D. EED

* Zaki Mubarak: A Critical Study.
                    By Dr. Mahmud Al Shihabi

* Summary of Saudi Arabian
                    Third Five year Development Plan

* Education in Saudi Arabia, A Model with Difference
                    By Dr. Abdulla Mohamed Al-Zaid.

* The Health of the Family in A Changing Arabia
                    By Dr. Zohair A. Sebai